Forthcoming Monographs

Holmes
**Diagnosis and Management of Seizures and
Epilepsy in Children**

Travis and Brouhard

Diabetes Mellitus in Children

Bluestone and Klein
Otitis Media in Infants and Children

Pediatric Orthopedics

Thomas S. Renshaw, M.D.

Director of Orthopaedic Surgery
Newington Children's Hospital
Newington, Connecticut

Volume 28 in the Series
MAJOR PROBLEMS IN CLINICAL PEDIATRICS

W. B. SAUNDERS COMPANY
Philadelphia London Toronto Mexico City Rio de Janeiro Sydney Tokyo Hong Kong

W. B. Saunders Company: West Washington Square
                          Philadelphia, PA   19105

Library of Congress Cataloging in Publication Data

Renshaw, Thomas S.

Pediatric orthopedics.

(Major problems in clinical pediatrics; v. 28)

1. Pediatric orthopedia.   I. Title.   II. Series.
   [DNLM: 1. Orthopedics—in infancy & childhood.
   W1 MA492N v.28/WS 270 R421p]

RD732.3.C48R46 1986   617'.3   85–19619

ISBN 0–7216–1179–6

Editor: Dana Dreibelbis
Designer: Patti Maddaloni
Production Manager: Laura Tarves
Illustration Coordinator: Walter Verbitski

Pediatric Orthopedics   ISBN   0–7216–1179–6

Last digit is the print number: 9   8   7   6   5   4   3   2

Foreword

Developmental and acquired orthopedic abnormalities unique to infants, children, and adolescents are fairly common problems encountered by physicians who care for this age group. For this reason, pediatric orthopedics is one of the topics more frequently requested by primary care physicians for inclusion in continuing education programs. That is why for some time we have wanted to include a volume on this subject in the MPCP monograph series.

Dr. Thomas Renshaw received his medical degree from Ohio State University. After an internship there, he spent two years as a surgeon in the Air Force, followed by four years of orthopedic training at the University of Michigan Medical Center. In 1974, he joined the orthopedic staff at Newington Children's Hospital, where he currently serves as Director of Orthopedics. Dr. Renshaw is the author of 25 articles and book chapters, and he has made more than a score of presentations throughout the country. He has a special interest in hip conditions and he is especially well known for his work in scoliosis. He has been among the leaders in devising and promoting screening programs for this condition.

This well-illustrated monograph is based on more than a decade of Dr. Renshaw's personal experience devoted entirely to the care of children at a large referral center for pediatric musculoskeletal conditions. It is written in a very readable style and contains succinct descriptions of all of the common and many of the uncommon orthopedic conditions as well as practical suggestions for their management.

MILTON MARKOWITZ, M.D.

Preface

Orthopedic conditions comprise a significant proportion (10% to 15%) of children's health problems. It is the author's hope that this text will be helpful to those who evaluate and treat these problems. This book is intended for use as a reference text by pediatricians; family physicians; pediatric, family practice, and orthopedic residents; nurse practitioners; and others who deal with common musculoskeletal problems in children. It is meant to be a practical guide, not a comprehensive treatise covering a broad spectrum of problems. Even the large two-volume pediatric orthopedic texts written specifically for pediatric orthopedic surgeons have great difficulty in accomplishing that.

The text is organized into five chapters covering the anatomic regions of the upper extremity, the spine, the hip, the lower extremity and knee, and the foot. These follow an introductory chapter that reviews the musculoskeletal examination. The final chapter discusses some of the more common generic problems and other special conditions seen in children's orthopedic practice. Clearly, the final chapter cannot be all inclusive. It covers such common conditions as cerebral palsy, myelomeningocele, other muscle disorders, and so forth. At the end of the book is a glossary of terms that have been extracted from the text and explained for quick reference.

The content of this book mostly reflects the author's ten years' experience at the Newington Children's Hospital, an institution that has provided pediatric orthopedic care for almost ninety years. Most of the material is factual and based on the Newington experience. Nevertheless, as with any single-author textbook, there must be some opinion, and some personal bias is inevitable. It is to be hoped that the bias has been kept to a minimum and that opinions have been clarified as such.

The illustrations for each chapter are mostly clinical photographs or radiographs, intended to cover almost all the described conditions. These are drawn from the wide spectrum of pediatric orthopedic conditions seen at the Newington Children's Hospital, a referral center for the northeastern United States. The references after each chapter are intended to provide referral to classic articles for specific conditions and also to some of the more recent articles that are either of general scope or more focused examples of current knowledge.

Acknowledgments

The author owes a major debt of gratitude to the Newington Children's Hospital and to those who maintain its high standards of care for children. The Hospital was established in 1898 and since then has been a resource of great value providing clinical health care, education for professionals and the public alike, and an environment for active clinical research. Those who have been employed by the Hospital or who donate their talents deserve major credit for providing the author with the opportunity to produce this book.

Although there are many distinguished physicians who have served as mentors, role models, and inspirations throughout the author's career, one who stands out most clearly is James M. Cary, M.D., a teacher of pediatric orthopedics with few peers. Many of his teachings are recognizable in this text. Much gratitude is also owed to my colleagues at the Newington Children's Hospital: Burr H. Curtis, M.D., John V. Banta, M.D., James C. Drennan, M.D., and James R. Gage, M.D., all dedicated pediatric orthopedic surgeons. Each has taught me a great deal. Newington's Director of Radiology, M. B. Ozonoff, M.D., has been of great help and guidance throughout the planning and preparation of this text.

There are many others without whose help this book would not have been possible. Particular thanks go to Barbara Dennis, who oversaw and coordinated all the multiple (and sometimes frustrating) changes in the text, the illustrations, the references, and the entire project. Special thanks also are due to Marianna Nelson, who helped with the final preparation of the text; to Jennifer Cox and her staff in the word processing section at Newington; and to Marion Shores, who provided the medical illustration. Gratitude is also in order to the staff of the photographic department at Newington Children's Hospital for their substantial work in preparing the clinical and radiographic illustrations.

Finally, my thanks to Milton Markowitz, M.D., and to Bill Lamsback and Dana Dreibelbis of the W. B. Saunders Company for their help throughout the preparation of this book.

The book is dedicated to children and to those who care for them.

Contents

Pediatric Orthopedic History Taking and Physical Examination

The examiner assesses a neonate, an infant, a child, or an adolescent for the purpose of evaluating signs or symptoms, or periodically to assure normality. Fortunately, the important skills of history taking and physical examination are easy to acquire and master. What is more difficult is acquiring the discipline to be thorough and to provide accurate follow-up of suspicious findings. Nevertheless, such an approach will enable one to identify potentially serious or even crippling conditions in childhood, many of which are subtle and may progress insidiously—particularly those involving the spine or the hip. As with most medical conditions, early detection of pediatric musculoskeletal disorders often avoids the need for complex treatment measures and leads to more favorable results.

HISTORY TAKING

Prenatal history is important regarding the mother's exposure to drugs or environmental toxins. Also important is the assessment of the intrauterine position, both during the pregnancy and at delivery. Congenital hip dysplasia has a higher incidence in breech-positioned babies. The mother's perception of decreased fetal activity may be the first sign of neuromuscular conditions such as arthrogryposis and spinal muscular atrophy. The order of birth is important, since it is known that congenital dysplasia of the hip is more likely to occur in first-born children. A history of oligohydramnios is often found with babies who have angular or torsional deformities of their legs or feet. Perinatal events such as the duration and character of labor, the type of delivery, Apgar scores, and other immediate postnatal factors should be assessed. These may have bearing on such conditions as cerebral palsy, torticollis, and Erb's palsy.

The assessment of developmental milestones is next. Children who are early walkers, are overweight, or have excessive physiologic bowleg (or a combination of these factors) are more likely to develop Blount's disease and other lower extremity problems. Achievement of developmental motor milestones may be delayed in neurologic disorders such as cerebral palsy and spinal muscular atrophy or in muscle diseases such as Duchenne's muscular dystrophy and congenital myopathies.

It is often useful to assess postural patterns, such as habitual sitting in the "W" or reversed tailor position or habitual sleeping in the knee-chest position with the feet tucked under the pelvis. Such prolonged posturing can explain the exaggeration or failure of improvement of foot and leg deformities.

Although the importance of assessing the regional anatomic structures relative to the presenting complaint is self-evident, it is noteworthy that referred pain is a common factor in misdiagnoses. Such conditions as slipped capital femoral epiphysis, Legg-Perthes disease, and tumors of the hip and pelvis often present with knee or anterior thigh pain. Similarly, spinal problems such as infections and tumors can present as abdominal, buttock, or lower extremity pain. It is important to remember that musculoskeletal problems may be associated with disease in other organs. For example, congenital spinal malformations are associated with renal anomalies (30% of cases) and cardiac malformations. Neural tube defects almost always have implications for dysfunction of the genitourinary and gastrointestinal tracts, and, conversely, abnormalities in the visceral organ systems should alert one to the possible presence of anomalies in the axial and appendicular skeleton.

After completing a review of systems and the past medical history, the history taker concludes with the family history. This is important because such conditions as dysplasia of the hip, spinal anomalies, ectrodactyly, flat feet, toe walking, metatarsus varus, and ligamentous laxity may have a familial or hereditary background. Finally, having a basic knowledge of genetics, consulting a current comprehensive textbook of genetic disorders, and gaining access to a good geneticist are most helpful in providing care to pediatric patients and their families.

PHYSICAL EXAMINATION

It almost goes without saying that throughout recorded medical history, those physicians who have been considered the greatest clinicians of their times have all been masters at the science of physical examination. Al-

though it is not always practical or convenient to perform a physical examination of sufficient thoroughness to detect asymptomatic problems, nevertheless, adopting this as a routine practice will set the physician-of-excellence apart from the average practitioner. This is true whether the reason for the examination is a routine screening or whether it is related to the focused evaluation of an episodic problem.

The physical examination begins with assessment of functional mobility, be it independent walking, sitting, achieved head control, or simply primitive reflexes in infants and in those who are neurologically impaired. Next comes an evaluation of gait, followed by assessment of the upper extremities, the spine, the hips, and the lower extremities, including the knees and feet (Fig. 1–1). Assessment of overall ligamentous laxity may also be important. Ligamentous laxity is assessed by looking at five particular areas. In the upper extremity, hyperextension of the metacarpophalangeal joints of the fingers

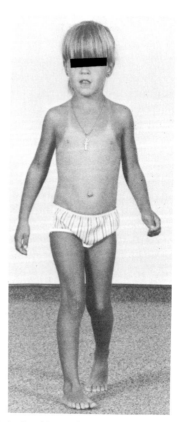

Figure 1–1. Intoeing gait secondary to femoral anteversion. Note the internal rotation of the entire right lower limb.

beyond 90 degrees is considered increased laxity. Recurvation of the elbows beyond 10 or 15 degrees also indicates hyperlaxity. Another upper extremity test is to place the wrist in maximum flexion and then attempt to approximate the thumb to the flexor surface of the forearm. When this can be done, the child's ligaments are lax. The other two findings are in the lower extremities, one being recurvation of the knees in excess of 10 to 15 degrees, and the other the ability to dorsiflex the foot to 60 degrees or beyond.

Evaluation of Gait

Toddlers have their own unique gait pattern, characterized by a wide base for stability, usually with external rotation of the legs and feet, and a flatfooted type of gait. This is the result of an immature central nervous system. The adult's smooth gait pattern is more complex but is much less energy-consuming. It usually develops between the ages of three and five years.

Many things can be learned simply by watching a child stand and walk (Fig. 1–2). The child should be clad only in underwear. First, note the angle of gait, which is the angle that the long axis of the foot makes with the direction the child is walking.

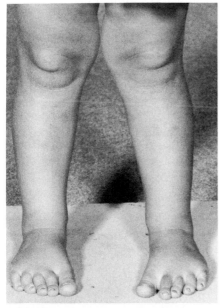

Figure 1–2. This two-year-old girl has excessive physiologic knock-knee and metatarsus varus.

Whereas most children will walk with a zero degree angle (feet pointing straight ahead), and inward variation beyond five to 10 degrees would be considered intoeing, and an outward variation beyond 10 to 15 degrees would be outtoeing. Note the stride length, which may be shortened in such conditions as hamstring tightness or spasticity of the muscles of the lower extremity, or in conditions in which pain in the lower back, hip, or leg is a component. Cadence may be slowed in conditions of weakness or pain or in other disorders.

The normal juvenile and adult gait cycle is measured from heel strike to heel strike on the same foot. During this cycle, the heel contacts the ground first; then the forefoot decelerates in a smooth fashion. Interference with deceleration caused by dorsiflexor weakness produces a drop-foot or slapping gait. After deceleration comes the midstance phase of "foot-flat," in which the weight is distributed throughout the foot, from the heel along the lateral border to the metatarsal heads. Deformities of the foot will decrease the weight-bearing surface area and will produce increased pressure in areas not designed to take such pressure. This ultimately leads to painful calluses and further deformity. Following the "foot-flat" phase, the last part of stance is toe-off, which is accompanied by hip and knee flexion designed to bring the limb forward. Then begins the swing phase of gait. Finally, the foot prepares to accept weight at heel strike, and another cycle begins.

The length of the stance phase should be observed. In normal walking, each limb is in stance phase for 60% of the gait cycle, and the remaining 40% of the cycle is swing phase. This gives a 20% overlap known as the period of double support. Stance phase is often shortened when there is pain accentuated by weight-bearing in the foot, knee, or hip.

Another common gait abnormality in children is abductor insufficiency, the so-called "abductor lurch" or trunk sway gait. This is caused by weakness of the hip abductor muscles, which normally maintain the pelvis in a level position during stance phase. With abductor weakness (usually associated with hip disease), the child is forced to lean toward the involved hip during stance phase in order to keep from losing balance (Fig. 1–3). This produces a lurch toward the affected side during ipsilateral stance phase.

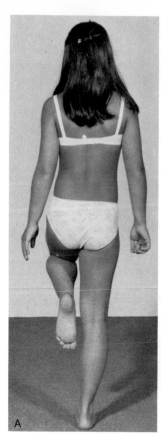
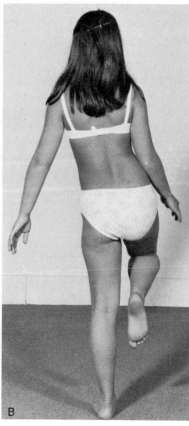

Figure 1–3. *A,* Normal balance when standing on the right leg. *B,* Abductor muscle weakness of the left hip causes leaning to the left to maintain balance and produces a lurch during walking.

Upper Extremity Evaluation

In infants and younger children, observation is a very valuable technique for upper extremity evaluation. One should look for pseudoparalysis or reluctance on the part of the infant to use the extremity. This can often be a sign of pain due to fractures, infections, or tumors, or it may be related to weakness secondary to cervical spine lesions or brachial plexus palsy. Upper extremity evaluation in infants and children should include assessment of the range of motion of the shoulder, elbow, wrist, and hand joints, and muscle testing to evaluate the size and strength of the various muscle groups of the shoulder and upper extremity. In cases of prior injury or infection, it is important to compare the upper extremities, noting if one is longer than the other.

It is sometimes difficult to evaluate the elbow in children. The normal neonate has a mild flexion contracture of the elbow, which disappears within a few weeks after birth.

Older children frequently traumatize their elbows and distal humeral regions. Clinical examination of a swollen, painful elbow can be very difficult, and radiographic examination is always essential. Obtaining comparison views of the contralateral normal elbow is of particular value when evaluating trauma. A helpful hint in examining the injured elbow is to remember that the medial humeral condyle, the lateral humeral condyle, and the olecranon process form a triangle. In the normal elbow, the lateral condyle is slightly more distal than the medial condyle (Fig. 1–4). If this relationship is disturbed when compared with that in the contralateral elbow, a fracture is likely. The radiographic interpretation of elbow injuries is often difficult and may require expert consultation.

The distal radius is a common site of fractures in children. One must assume that a fracture is present if there is definite tenderness over the distal radius or the wrist, regardless of the radiographic findings. Microfractures do occur, and when in doubt,

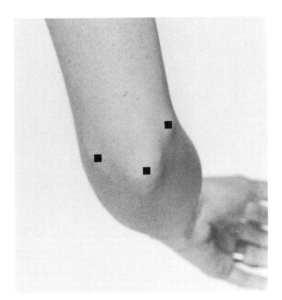

Figure 1–4. A normal left elbow. Note that the lateral humeral condyle is slightly distal to the medial condyle.

one is well advised to protect the extremity in a splint or cast and later to reevaluate the situation.

Evaluation of The Spine

Physical evaluation of the cervical spine begins by observing for torticollis and then asking the patient to demonstrate the range of motion of the neck. This includes flexion, extension, lateral bending, and lateral rotation to each side. In infants and children who are too young to cooperate, passive range of motion can be evaluated while the child lies on a parent's lap. This should always be done with great care and gentleness, the examiner being ready to stop immediately should the patient have any symptoms of pain or paresthesia or signs of muscle spasm. When in doubt, appropriate radiographic evaluation should be obtained first. There have been reported cases of neurologic injury or damage to the vertebral arteries, or both, due to forceful manipulation of the cervical spine.

Examination of the neck also includes palpation for masses and evaluation of sternocleidomastoid muscle tightness in cases of torticollis. This muscle is at its maximum length when the head is tilted away from the side being tested and is rotated maximally toward the ipsilateral side. Maximum slack in the sternomastoid occurs when the head is tilted toward the ipsilateral side and rotated toward the contralateral side. This can be easily demonstrated by placing your thumb on the medial end of your own clavicle with your long finger on your mastoid and reproducing these maneuvers. All cases of torticollis should be radiographically evaluated to rule out anomalies of the spinal column.

Examination of the thoracic and lumbar spine should be done by inspection and then palpation. Standing posture should be observed, including any signs of scoliosis, hyperkyphosis, or hyperlordosis (Fig. 1–5). Note should be made whether or not there is a skin disorder over the spine, which may indicate a congenital spinal or neurologic anomaly. Such pathologic conditions include hemangiomata, soft or cystic masses, dimples, sinus tracts, and areas of hypertrichosis. With the patient in the forward bending position, the spine should be observed from the front, the back, and the side to look for further spinal deformity. The patient should then demonstrate active range of motion of the spine, which should be smooth and rhythmic. During this maneuver, palpation will identify muscle spasm or atrophy.

Neurologic evaluation completes the examination of the spine. This includes muscle testing in the upper and lower extremities; sensory evaluation; assessment of deep tendon reflexes; testing for pathologic reflexes; and looking for limb length inequality, atrophy, or foot deformity. A history of bowel or bladder dysfunction may also indicate an intraspinal lesion.

Hip Evaluation

It cannot be overstated that all neonates and infants should undergo repeated evaluations of their hips to rule out congenital dysplasia. This evaluation is discussed in Chapter 4. Evaluation for hip problems in older children begins with assessment of gait, noting such findings as a positive Trendelenburg sign, an abductor lurch, or an antalgic gait. Next, the lower limb lengths are measured, and any pelvic obliquity is noted. This is best detected by placing one's hands on the iliac crests and noting their levels. Another reliable means is to identify the dimples present over the sacroiliac joints of most patients. If these are symmetric and at the same height, pelvic obliquity is absent. Hip muscle

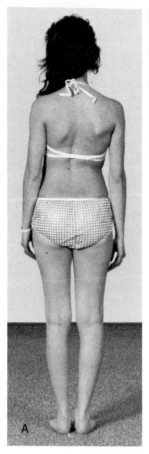

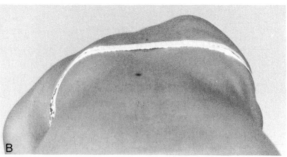

Figure 1–5. *A*, This girl has scoliosis. When she is viewed from the back, there is a notable difference in scapula heights and apparent flattening of the left waistline. *B*, When the patient bends forward (the Adams test), a large right rib prominence is seen.

strength should be tested, both by the Trendelenburg test and also by having the patient flex, extend, adduct, abduct, and rotate the hip against the examiner's resistance.

The range of hip motion in flexion and extension is tested with the patient in the supine position. To test for hip flexion contractures, both hips should be flexed maximally. Then the patient should hold one thigh in that position with both hands while the examiner gently brings the other hip into as much extension as possible. This maneuver, the Thomas test, will stabilize the pelvis and prevent lumbar lordosis from masking a hip flexion contracture (Fig. 1–6). Hip abduction and adduction can also be tested with the patient recumbent. Abductor muscle strength is noted with the patient in the sidelying position. One must be sure that the pelvis is truly vertical, since patients will try to compensate for weak abductors by rolling their pelvis into posterior obliquity and then using their hip flexors as spurious abductors.

Hip rotation must be measured with the patient in the prone position, which assures extension of the hips and a tightened anterior hip joint capsule. Otherwise, with a lax capsule, artificially increased rotation may be noted as the femoral head cams or subluxes from the acetabulum. In infants and young children, external rotation normally exceeds internal rotation. In older children and adults, internal and external rotation are approximately equal. Patients who demonstrate excessive internal rotation (greater than 60 degrees) are likely to have excessive femoral anteversion (Fig. 1–7), whereas excessive external rotation may indicate femoral retroversion (Fig. 1–8).

Subtle signs of hip disease are often detectable by having the patient lie supine and completely relax the lower extremities. Then, by gently rolling the limb back and forth, one can detect subtle loss of rotation, which may be an indicator of synovitis or an irritable hip. This test is particularly sensitive in picking up early cases of Legg-Perthes disease and slipped capital femoral epiphysis. In chil-

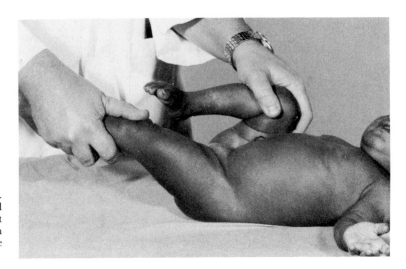

Figure 1–6. The Thomas test. When the pelvis is stabilized and the lumbar spine is flattened out by flexing the right hip, a flexion contracture of the left hip can be detected.

dren who are able to relax completely, the femoral head can be palpated both anteriorly and posteriorly. This can help to confirm local tenderness or synovitis.

Finally, it is imperative to remember that hip pain is frequently referred to the anterolateral thigh or the anterior knee, or both. It is essential to assess the condition of the hip, with both clinical and radiographic examinations, in any patient who presents with pain from the region of the waistline down to and including the knee.

Lower Extremity Evaluation

Examination of the lower extremity includes observing the child's gait, measuring limb lengths, assessing muscle bulk or atrophy (or both), noting joint motion ranges, and testing for gross muscle strength of the hip, thigh, and leg muscles. The angle of the knee (tibiofemoral angle) can be assessed on clinical examination, measured with a protractor, documented with photographs, or assessed more precisely by measuring the angle on a standing radiograph taken with the child's feet pointing straight ahead. Palpation for assessment of areas of inflammation, potential tumors, or thrombophlebitis may also be important. Next, one can evaluate tibial torsion by estimating the axis of knee flexion and extension and comparing this with the axis of ankle flexion and extension, as well as with the bimalleolar axis of the ankle joint (Fig. 1–9). The normal infant has zero to 20 degrees of internal tibial torsion, which changes to approximately 20 de-

grees (plus or minus 15) of external tibial torsion by the end of growth. Most of this growth rotation is accomplished by the age of seven years.

Knee Examination

Knee examination also begins with observation of the patient's gait, limb lengths, and thigh and calf circumference. Many pathologic conditions affecting the knee joint are accompanied by thigh atrophy and, often, calf atrophy. One should look and palpate for effusion of the knee joint and synovitis, and one should evaluate the active range of motion of the knee and the strength of the thigh and calf muscles. Knee ligament stability should be evaluated by using specific tests to detect instability of the cruciate, collateral, and capsular ligaments. The retropatellar fat pad should be palpated for swelling or tenderness. Compression tests for meniscus integrity are also important.

Finally, the patellofemoral joint should be examined by looking for patella alta or patella baja, noting the "Q" angle and testing for hypermobility of the patella. By displacing the patella both medially and laterally with the knee extended and the quadriceps relaxed, the surfaces of the patellar facet joints can be palpated for tenderness or irregularities. The Fairbank test (lateral displacement) for "patellar apprehension" is also valuable in cases of a subluxing or dislocating patella. Patellofemoral crepitus or tenderness is detected with the quadriceps relaxed. The patella is compressed manually

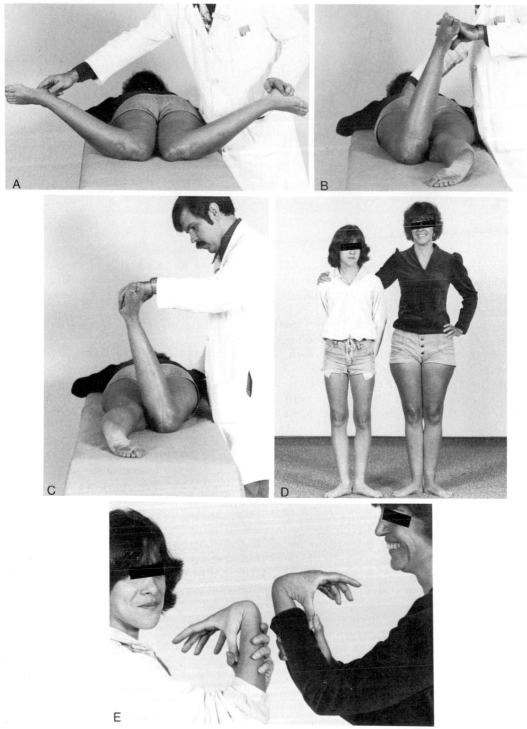

Figure 1–7. *A*, Femoral anteversion in an adult female. There is approximately 70 degrees of internal hip rotation bilaterally. *B* and *C*, External rotation is about 10 degrees on each side. Note surgical scars on each knee due to patellar re-alignment procedures. *D* and *E*, Her daughter demonstrated similar findings, as well as ligamentous laxity. She was treated with prophylactic femoral derotation osteotomies.

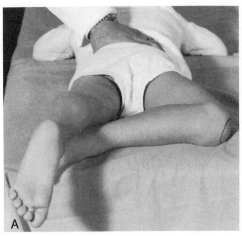 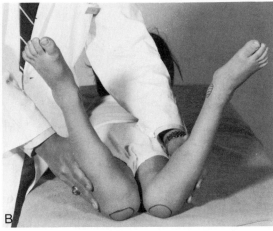

Figure 1–8. Excessive (90 degrees) external hip rotation in a three-year-old boy. *B*, Internal hip rotation in the same child was limited to about 30 degrees. Radiographic examination revealed femoral retroversion.

against the front of the femur and moved up and down and back and forth. It is also detectable by having the patient maximally contract the relaxed quadriceps while the patella is being compressed. Further diag-

nostic studies such as arthrography or arthroscopy are sometimes indicated.

Foot Evaluation

A knowledge of normal foot development is essential in interpreting an evaluation of the foot. The foot examination should include observation of the patient's barefoot gait for the angle of gait and the stability of the foot during stance phase. While observing gait, it is helpful to notice whether the abductor hallucis muscle is overactive. This is frequently the case in infants and toddlers who toe-in.

One then observes the skin and vascular status of the foot and examines for ankle, tarsal, metatarsal, and toe joint flexibility and motion. Observing the patient standing barefoot on a firm surface facilitates the assessment of heel varus or valgus, the height of the longitudinal medial arch, and the presence or absence of cavus. Whether there is claw toe deformity, hallux valgus deformity, or other toe problems should also be noted.

Radiographs of the foot should usually be taken with the patient standing. The films ordered should include an anteroposterior (AP) view of both feet while bearing the patient's weight and a lateral view of each foot in neutral or maximum dorsiflexion. With the feet in these positions, heel cord tightness and the relationship of the talus to the os calcis can be more accurately assessed. Oblique views are useful in detecting congenital foot anomalies such as tarsal coalitions (Fig. 1–10).

Figure 1–9. Internal tibial torsion—right greater than left. With knees facing forward, the ankle is rotated inward.

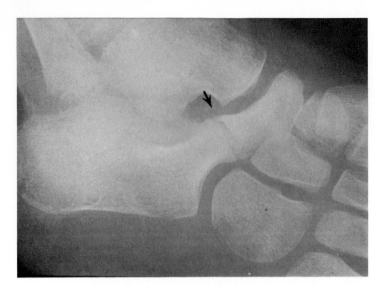

Figure 1–10. Oblique radiograph demonstrating incomplete calcaneonavicular coalition.

References

Blount WP: Fractures in Children. Baltimore, Williams and Wilkins, 1954.

Coleman SS: Complex Foot Deformities in Children. Philadelphia, Lea and Febiger, 1983.

Harris NH: Postgraduate Textbook of Clinical Orthopaedics. Bristol, John Wright and Sons Ltd, 1983.

Hensinger RN and Jones ET: Neonatal Orthopaedics. New York, Grune and Stratton Inc, 1981.

Inman VT: Human Walking. Baltimore, Williams and Wilkins, 1978.

Lovell WW and Winter RB: Pediatric Orthopaedics. Philadelphia, JB Lippincott Co, 1978.

Moe JH et al.: Scoliosis and Other Spinal Deformities. Philadelphia, WB Saunders Co, 1978.

Ozonoff MB: Pediatric Orthopedic Radiology. Philadelphia, WB Saunders Co, 1979.

Rang M: Children's Fractures. Philadelphia, JB Lippincott Co, 1974.

Scoles PV: Pediatric Orthopedics in Clinical Practice. Chicago, Year Book Medical Publishers, Inc, 1982.

Sharrard WJW: Pediatric Orthopaedics and Fractures, 2nd ed. Oxford, Blackwell Scientific Publications, 1979.

Sutherland DH et al.: The development of mature gait. J Bone Joint Surg 62A:336, 1980.

Tachdjian, MO: Pediatric Orthopedics. Philadelphia, WB Saunders Co, 1972.

2

The Upper Extremity

Most upper extremity problems are quickly and easily recognized by children, parents, grandparents, well-meaning friends, and all health care providers. Congenital and traumatic problems are common; both occur in the upper limb more often than in the lower extremity.

THE HAND

Syndactyly

This condition, sometimes called "webbed fingers," is one of the most common congenital abnormalities of the upper extremity. The severity of involvement varies from minimal proximal bridging between adjacent fingers to complete webbing of the entire hand, the so-called "mitten hand." The more severe the syndactyly, the more likely there are to be underlying bony anomalies as well. The most common site of syndactyly is between the long and ring fingers, followed by the ring and small fingers, the long and index fingers, and the thumb and index finger, in decreasing order of occurrence (Fig. 2–1).

Treatment is based upon the severity of the webbing and the presence or absence of underlying bone abnormalities. If only two fingers are involved and the bone structure is normal, then function will be excellent. In that instance correction can wait until the child is three or four years old, since the larger hand is technically easier to correct. With multiple fingers involved or significant

bony involvement, function may deteriorate with growth, and earlier correction should be considered. The major risk of correction is vascular compromise in a finger. Severe syndactyly may accompany more general conditions such as Streeter's dysplasia, Poland's syndrome, or Apert's syndrome.

Polydactyly

Supernumerary digits occur more commonly in blacks than in Caucasians and can vary markedly in size and significance. The most common type is a small, rudimentary, floppy appendage or skin tag on either the radial or the ulnar side of the hand. This is best treated in the newborn period with simple but careful surgical excision with the patient under local anesthesia. This is far more professional and humane than the older practice of ligation of the pedicle.

The other end of the polydactyly spectrum is a completely duplicated normal-appearing digit, giving a fully functional six-fingered hand. This may be hereditary, as seen in the Ellis-van Creveld syndrome. Most instances of polydactyly fall somewhere between the two extremes. Often, only the distal phalanx is duplicated, as commonly seen in the thumb.

For the more involved cases, therapeutic decisions should be based not only on cosmetic appearance but also on function. For this reason, it is best to defer a decision until the child is old enough for an accurate eval-

11

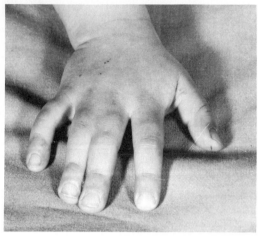

Figure 2–1. Partial syndactyly of the long and ring fingers of the right hand.

uation of the hand's fine motor function to be done. Definitive treatment should be carried out before the beginning of nursery school or kindergarten, since deformed hands are readily apparent to all.

Macrodactyly

Localized enlargement of one or more digits may occur either as an idiopathic deformity that maintains its proportionate enlargement throughout growth and development, or as a progressively enlarging abnormality produced by a pathologic process such as neurofibromatosis or vascular or lymphatic anomalies (Fig. 2–2). When multiple digits are involved, they are usually adjacent.

Surgical treatment of this condition yields less than optimal results in most cases. Operations designed to reduce the size of the finger include epiphyseal arrests and defatting procedures. With the progressively increasing type and with single digit involvement, amputation of the ray, including the metacarpal, may be the best procedure. The best timing of surgery is after the neonatal period.

Clinodactyly

Clinodactyly, or "curved finger," occurs most commonly in the small finger but also frequently involves the index finger (Fig. 2–3). The condition is usually bilateral and is most often the result of unequal growth of the epiphysis of the middle phalanx. Milder cases are best treated with reassurance. More severe deformities may be corrected by osteotomy, done at or after the end of the growth period.

Kirner's Deformity

Kirner's deformity is curving of the distal phalanx of the little finger in a radial and palmar direction (Fig. 2–4). Its onset is after age seven, and it is more common in girls. Most cases are asymptomatic, do not have a functional deficit, and require no treatment. Splinting is effective for painful cases. Osteotomy is successful but rarely necessary.

Figure 2–2. Idiopathic macrodactyly of the right thumb.

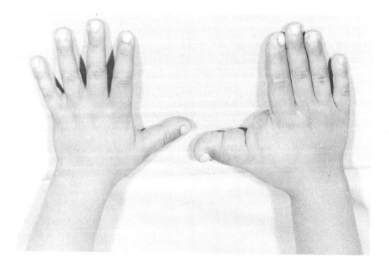

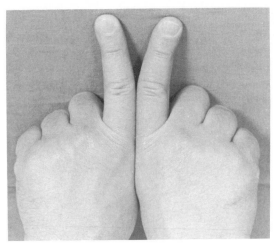

Figure 2–3. Clinodactyly of the index fingers.

Camptodactyly

This common condition is a flexion contracture of the proximal interphalangeal joint, usually of the small finger (Fig. 2–5). It

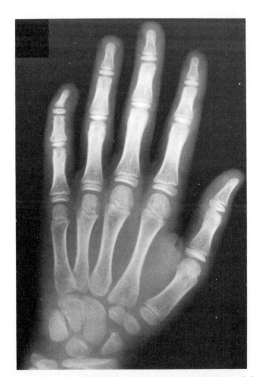

Figure 2–4. Kirner's deformity of the little finger of the left hand. Note the radial deviation of the distal phalanx.

is a congenital anomaly not related to trauma or any other known cause and may be inherited as an autosomal dominant trait. Multiple fingers may be involved. When this is the case, one should look for more generalized conditions such as congenital contractural arachnodactyly, arthrogryposis multiplex congenita, or one of the bone dysplasias.

The results of early splinting are usually unsatisfactory. It is best to treat contractures of less than 45 degrees with reassurance and to reserve appropriate soft tissue release and tendon surgery for more severely involved fingers.

Ectrodactyly (Lobster-Claw Hand)

This is an autosomal dominant condition characterized by the absence of central rays, often the middle or ring finger, with absent or rudimentary metacarpals (Fig. 2–6). It may be bilateral in the upper extremity and may be associated with similar deformities of the feet. Despite the rather grotesque appearance of the hand, function is usually quite good. The decision to improve the cosmetic appearance through narrowing of the cleft should be made by an experienced hand surgeon with the best of surgical judgment, in order not to compromise function.

Symphalangism

Symphalangism is a congenital synostosis of the proximal interphalangeal joint and may occur in isolation or in multiple fingers (Fig. 2–7). It is recognized in the newborn as stiffness and is sometimes termed the "single-joint finger." It is important to rule out camptodactyly. The only treatment for symphalangism is angulation osteotomy to enable better functional grip, although this is rarely necessary.

Trigger Thumb

This condition is usually detected in midinfancy, when it is noted that the child is unable to extend fully the interphalangeal joint of the thumb. Most often there is a palpable nodule or fusiform enlargement along the flexor tendon in the region of the metacarpophalangeal joint, which is adaptive and is secondary to a congenital constriction in the fibrous sheath of the flexor pollicis longus

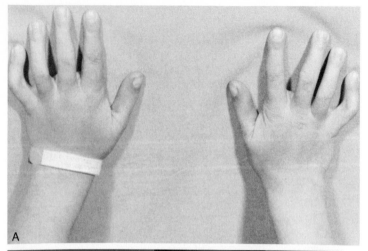

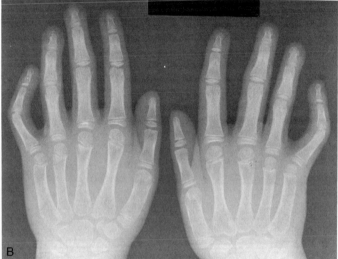

Figure 2–5. Clinical *(A)* and radiographic *(B)* views of camptodactyly involving the little fingers.

Figure 2–6. Ectrodactyly involving both hands. This patient had useful opposition of both thumb structures and functioned quite well without reconstructive surgery.

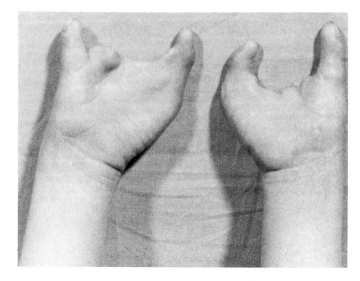

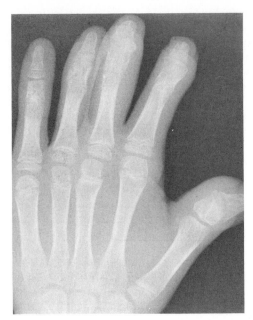

Figure 2–7. Symphalangism involving all digits of the hand.

tendon. If the stenosis is sufficiently tight, the interphalangeal joint appears to be fixed in flexion. If there is less stenosis, then passive extension of the joint causes a sudden snapping release as the enlargement passes through the tight area, the so-called "triggering" phenomenon. The differential diagnosis of trigger thumb includes the normal flexed thumb-in-palm position of the neonate, neuromuscular disease with joint contracture, and congenital absence of the thumb's extensor tendons.

When trigger thumb is diagnosed in early infancy, nonsurgical treatment is worthy of trial. This consists of gentle passive stretching and then splinting of the thumb in extension at the interphalangeal joint. One should not delay surgical correction beyond the age of six months, however, since in older children a permanent contracture may develop. Surgical treatment consists of simple longitudinal release of the constriction in the fibrous tendon sheath through a small transverse skin incision.

Triphalangeal Thumb

This is a rare anomaly, often inherited by autosomal dominant transmission. The diagnosis is usually made when the thumb is noted to be excessively long. The thumb may or may not have abnormal angulation. One should look for associated upper extremity anomalies such as the Holt-Oram syndrome. The treatment of a triphalangeal thumb depends upon its length, angular deformity, and joint stability. Shortening or fusion procedures, or both, may be indicated for sufficiently deformed cases.

Fractures and Dislocations

Fractures of the phalanges in children commonly occur through either the growth plate or the shaft of the bone (Fig. 2–8). Precision is necessary in their reduction to prevent residual angulatory or rotatory deformity, which can significantly interfere with function. Fractures that involve articular surfaces require perfect reduction with restoration of an anatomic joint surface. A digital fracture that cannot be adequately reduced by closed means should be treated with open reduction and internal fixation. Regardless of treatment, the usual period of immobili-

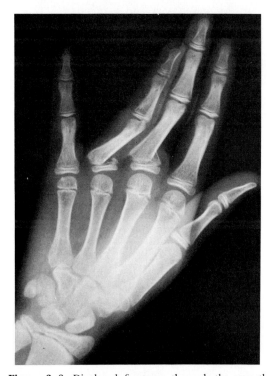

Figure 2–8. Displaced fractures through the growth plates at the base of the proximal phalanges of the long and ring finger of the left hand.

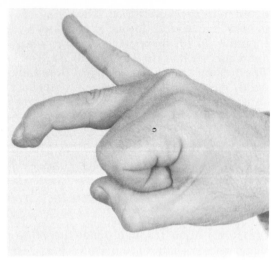

Figure 2–9. An untreated mallet finger. Despite persistent deformity, there was no significant functional loss.

zation for children's finger fractures is three to four weeks.

A common phalangeal fracture is the "mallet finger" caused by rupture of the extensor tendon or fracture of the dorsal base of the distal phalanx (Fig. 2–9). Treatment is splinting the distal joint in hyperextension.

The most common metacarpal fracture in children and adolescents is fracture of the neck of the fifth metacarpal, often sustained in fist-fighting (Fig. 2–10). The usual presentation is pain and swelling proximal to the head of the fifth metacarpal. Radiographic examination reveals a dorsally angulated, transverse fracture with depression volarly of the metacarpal head. Because of the mobility at the carpometacarpal joint of the fifth ray, perfect reduction is unnecessary, and simple closed reduction with immobilization for three weeks is all that is required in most cases.

Dislocations of interphalangeal joints are extremely uncommon in children, owing to the strength of the ligaments and the relative weakness of the epiphyseal plates. Most injuries that appear to be dislocations are, in reality, epiphyseal plate fractures. The most common dislocation in a child's hand occurs at the metacarpophalangeal joint of the thumb (Fig. 2–11). This is usually caused by a hyperextension injury in which the proximal phalanx dislocates dorsally and the metacarpal head "buttonholes" through a longi-

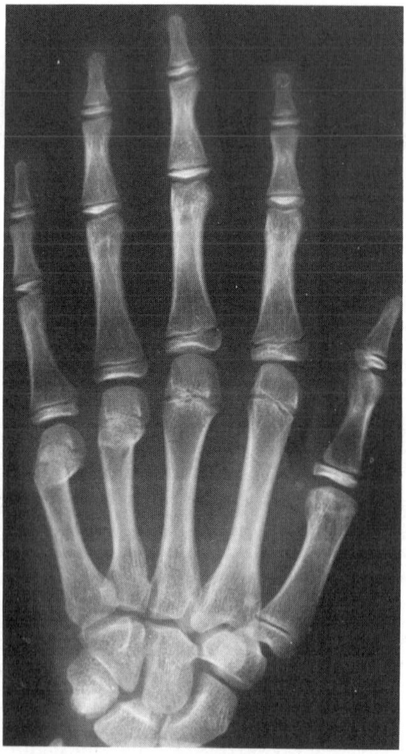

Figure 2–10. Volar and radially displaced fractures of the necks of the distal left fourth and fifth metacarpals. This is the so-called "Boxer's fracture."

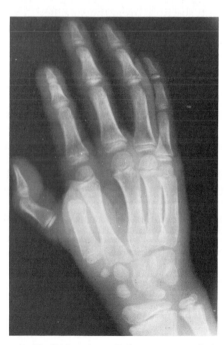

Figure 2–11. Dislocation of the metacarpophalangeal joint of the right thumb caused by hyperextension while playing football.

tudinal tear in the volar capsule. This may prevent satisfactory reduction by closed means and may require open reduction and soft tissue repair. Dislocations of other metacarpophalangeal joints may also be unreducible by closed means, because the volar plate frequently becomes trapped between the articular surfaces. In these instances, open reduction is required.

CONGENITAL LIMB DEFICIENCIES

Congenital deficiencies of parts of a limb can be classified very broadly into transverse (either segmental or complete absence distal to a transverse plane) or longitudinal types (only part of the limb distal to a given plane is absent). Under the categories of transverse and longitudinal there are two classifications: intercalary (a segmental deficit with the distal part intact, whether abnormal or normal) and terminal (all parts absent distal to a given point). The more common congenital deficiencies in the upper limb are absence of the radius and, less often, absence of the ulna.

Congenital Deficiency of the Radius

This condition, also known as "radial club hand," is a longitudinal deficiency and may be intercalary or terminal (Fig. 2–12). In slightly more than half the patients, it is a terminal longitudinal deficiency with complete absence of the radius and the thumb ray. In the remainder of the cases, there may be a hypoplastic proximal radius present with or without a hypoplastic thumb. The deficiency is bilateral in almost 50% of the children.

In assessing radial deficits, it is important to know that other congenital anomalies are frequently present. In bilateral cases, almost all patients will have other anomalies. The most common system involved is the genitourinary system, followed by the spine and then the gastrointestinal tract. Cardiac defects and a congenital type of thrombocytopenia have also been associated with radial deficits. Congenital radial deficiency is also a recognized component of the VATER syndrome (characterized by abnormalities of the Vertebrae, Anus [imperforate], Tracheo-Esophageal region, and Radius).

The clinical presentation of radial deficiency is a shortened forearm with bowing of

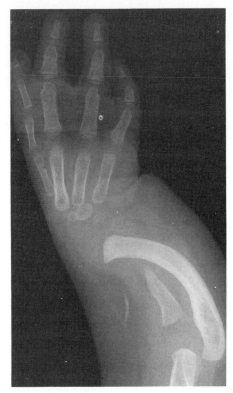

Figure 2–12. Congenital deficiency of the radius. Note bowing of the ulna and absence of the thumb ray.

the ulna, convex to the ulnar side and posteriorly. Elbow motion is usually limited. The thumb is absent or hypoplastic, and the hand deviates in a radial direction which, untreated, is progressive with growth, often exceeding 90 degrees. Abnormalities may exist in the neurovascular structures, the radial nerve often being absent and the radial artery variably so. A fibrous anlage of the missing radius may be palpable.

The management of this condition consists of gentle passive stretching exercises and the use of serial casts or splints, beginning in the newborn nursery. These are utilized in an attempt either to maintain the hand in a position of centralization in line with the distal ulna or to correct it into such a position. In unilateral cases, centralization by surgical means is usually required, in which the carpus is fixed to the distal ulna. This is best done in later infancy or early childhood. Still later, improved function may be obtained in selected cases by pollicization of the index finger. In bilateral cases, function is usually quite good, and the decision whether to attempt to centralize one or both of the hands

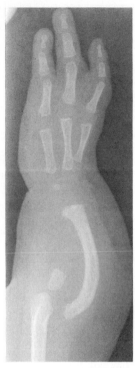

Figure 2–13. Congenital ulnar hemimelia. Note bowing of the radius.

should be left to an experienced pediatric hand surgeon.

Congenital Deficiency of the Ulna

This condition is far less common than radial deficiency. It is a longitudinal and usually terminal deficiency that is rarely complete, the usual finding being a hypoplastic proximal ulna that articulates with the humerus in some fashion (Fig. 2–13). Bilaterality is extremely rare in ulnar deficiency. The association of other congenital anomalies with this disorder is not common, but scoliosis and mandibular and fibular deformities have been reported.

The clinical presentation of ulnar deficiency is shortening of the forearm and bowing of the radius. The ulnar rays are usually absent but may be hypoplastic or otherwise abnormal. The radial head is often dislocated from the humerus. The wrist joint is usually stable and relatively normal, although ulnar deviation of the hand, sometimes of substantial magnitude, is common. The treatment of this condition is surgically to produce a "single-bone forearm."

THE CONGENITAL BAND SYNDROME (STREETER'S DYSPLASIA)

Annular constricting bands noted at birth may occur in any extremity and can vary from shallow transverse grooves to those causing near-complete or complete amputation (Fig. 2–14). When bilateral, they are usually asymmetric. Anomalies distal to the bands are common and include syndactyly, partial limb deficits, and occasionally edema or even ischemia. There is a high association with clubfoot, particularly with lower extremity bands.

The cause of congenital bands is not specifically known, but the most widely accepted theory is the presence of amniotic bands or other placental disorders associated with prenatal hemorrhages in the extremities. Although some have postulated embryonic defects to be the cause, this is not a hereditary condition, and most people believe that it is the result of abnormalities of the intrauterine environment.

Treatment depends upon the severity of the condition. Mild grooves do not need treatment. Bands that cause vascular or lymphatic obstruction or that are severely deforming should be released down to and including the fascia of the limb, followed by Z-plasty type closure. Such procedures should be staged so that no more than 60% of the band is excised at the first stage; otherwise, the risk of further lymphatic or vascular compromise may be increased.

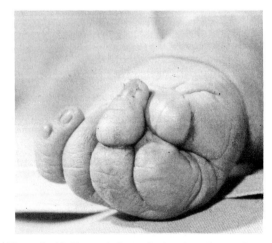

Figure 2–14. Congenital annular band syndrome (Streeter's dysplasia) involving the left hand.

When lesions having the appearance of congenital bands appear to arise de novo after birth, one should look very closely for a thin twisted strand of hair or thread that could be producing the lesion. Prompt release of this acquired constriction is essential.

RADIOULNAR SYNOSTOSIS

Radioulnar synostosis is a congenital fusion of the radius and ulna, usually at their proximal ends (Fig. 2–15). The condition is probably caused by the failure of complete division of the radius and ulna from their precursor block of mesenchymal tissue. Normally, separation begins distally and proceeds proximally. The condition occurs approximately equally in both sexes. About 50% of the cases are bilateral. The diagnosis is usually made in mid or late childhood, since the infant and young child have not yet developed the fine motor control required for precise forearm rotation. Although no forearm rotation is possible with this condition, the shoulder and the wrist are excellent at compensating for it.

In younger children, the connecting bar may be completely cartilaginous and therefore radiolucent. Most cases have associated dislocation or subluxation of the head of the radius. Bowing of the radius is also seen. This condition may be associated with other anomalies of the wrist and hand and has also

been reported in association with chromosomal abnormalities.

The treatment of radioulnar synostosis is reassurance, since significant interference with function is rare. Attempts to divide the synostosis and establish forearm rotation are unsuccessful. Occasionally, osteotomy of the bones of the forearm may be necessary to improve the position of the hand for grasping.

MADELUNG'S DEFORMITY

This is a deformity of the distal radius and ulna and is usually not noted until late childhood or adolescence. It is much more common in females and is bilateral in two thirds of cases. The clinical presentation is a shortened radius with bowing convex to the radial side, and a dorsally displaced and very prominent distal ulna (Fig. 2–16). The cause of Madelung's deformity is a genetic abnormality, often an autosomal dominant trait, which results in markedly impaired growth or even premature fusion of the ulnar and volar quadrant of the distal radial growth plate. There is significant volar angulation of the distal radius and wrist joint.

The condition may be associated with dyschondrosteosis, a bone dysplasia more common in females. The dysplasia results in short stature, with particular shortening in the tibial regions as well as in the forearms. Made-

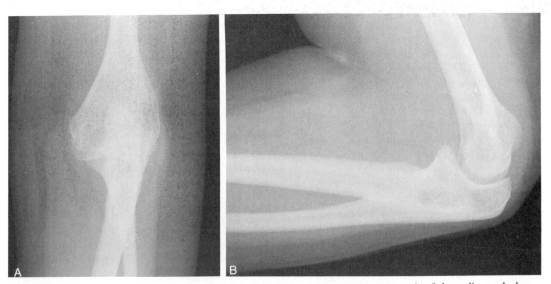

Figure 2–15. AP *(A)* and lateral *(B)* views of the right elbow demonstrating synostosis of the radius and ulna.

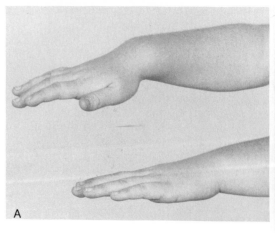
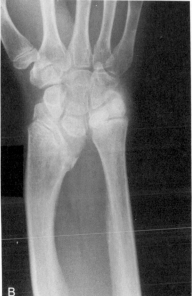

Figure 2–16. *A,* Madelung's deformity of the right forearm and wrist. *B,* Note the fusion of the distal radius growth plate laterally.

lung's deformity can also occur as an isolated case when there is no prior knowledge of genetic involvement.

Madelung's deformity is treated by completing the arrest of the growth plate of the distal radius, combined with corrective osteotomy through the metaphysis of the radius and excision of the distal ulna. The results of this treatment are generally quite good in terms of relief of pain and deformity, but there is little improvement of grip strength or range of motion.

WRIST FRACTURES

While traumatic injuries of the distal forearm are extremely common in children, fractures of the carpal bones are not. The most common carpal fracture in this age group is the scaphoid (navicular) fracture, an injury seen in adolescents, but more commonly in adults (Fig. 2–17). This is usually produced by a fall onto the outstretched thenar eminence with the wrist in dorsiflexion. The patient presents with pain and tenderness over the scaphoid bone, just distal to the radial styloid. Swelling is minimal, and not infrequently radiographs initially show negative findings. Special views are often necessary, including oblique views or magnification views, or both. Scaphoid fractures are notoriously slow to heal, require prolonged immobilization, and may result in nonunion and

therefore require surgical intervention. Because this fracture may be such a problem, it is best to assume that there is no such thing as a wrist sprain. If radiographs initially show

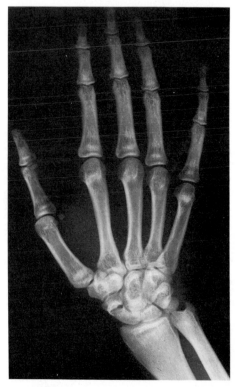

Figure 2–17. Fracture of the carpal scaphoid bone in an adolescent whose skeleton is mature.

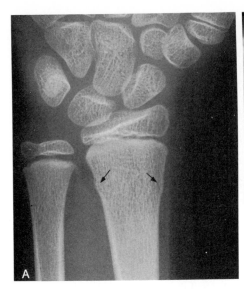

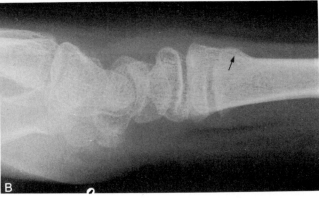

Figure 2–18. *A* and *B*, Torus fracture of the distal radius.

negative findings, the prudent physician will immobilize a traumatized wrist for 10 days and then repeat the radiographic studies. At that time, if there is a fracture present, bone resorption at the fracture site should be evident.

Although technically not fractures of the wrist, fractures through the distal radial growth plate or distal radial metaphysis are among the most common pediatric fractures.

The torus fracture of the distal radius or ulna, or both, is the result of a fall onto the outstretched hand. Subsequently, pain, tenderness, and usually mild swelling are seen in the distal radial metaphyseal region. Radiographs show a buckle or crease in the cortex of the bone and an area of increased density, which appears as a transverse linear extension from the cortical irregularity (Fig. 2–18). These are stable fractures, but since

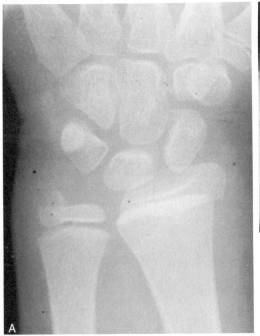

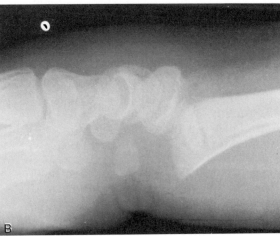

Figure 2–19. AP *(A)* and lateral *(B)* views of the left wrist showing a dorsally displaced fracture through the growth plate of the distal radius. Note that the distal ulna is intact.

the bone is weakened, they require protection in a short-arm cast for two to three weeks. This is also necessary for comfort.

Fractures through the distal radial growth plate are also quite common and may result in significant displacement of the epiphysis, often with a small triangular metaphyseal fragment (Fig. 2–19). The deformity is just proximal to the wrist joint, and there may be significant displacement and swelling. Reduction is quite simple, and further appropriate treatment consists of use of a long-arm splint or cast to hold the wrist in a position that will maintain stability. Immobilization continues three to six weeks depending upon the age of the child, the longer time being reserved for adolescents.

Fractures of the distal radius and ulna in the metaphyseal region that are displaced or angulated in the plane of wrist flexion and extension must be reduced, but they have some capacity to be remodeled. Deformity not in the plane of motion does not remodel well and must be corrected at the time of initial treatment.

FOREARM FRACTURES

Forearm fractures in the midshaft of the radius and ulna in children require substantial force to produce, and, therefore, careful attention to the soft tissues of the forearm is mandatory, lest an occult compartment syndrome and subsequent Volkmann's ischemic contracture result. Fractures that are incomplete or "greenstick," or fractures that involve one bone associated with only a bending or plastic deformity of the other are notoriously deceptive. In nearly all cases, proper treatment consists of completing the fracture of both bones so that reduction without angulation or rotatory deformity can be accomplished (Fig. 2–20). Complete fractures through both bones associated with displacement or deformity require expert closed reduction. Remodeling is much less predictable in the midshaft region, and fractures with rotatory or medial or lateral deformity may not be satisfactorily remodeled.

The treatment of forearm fractures, after acceptable reduction, is use of a long-arm cast for at least six weeks and then perhaps further protection, depending upon the appearance of the healing at that time. There is almost never any indication for use of open

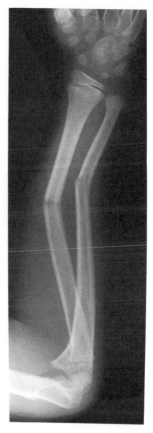

Figure 2–20. Angulated fractures of the shafts of the radius and ulna. Note the incomplete fracture of the ulna. This is best managed by completing the fracture, performing closed reduction, and immobilizing the fractures in a long arm cast until healing has occurred.

reduction and internal fixation of a forearm fracture in a child.

The Monteggia fracture is an angulated fracture of the proximal ulna with associated dislocation of the radius at the elbow (Fig. 2–21). This dislocation may be difficult to detect in the swollen elbows of young children when the radial head is still cartilaginous or when spontaneous total or partial reduction has occurred. Closed reduction of the fracture is usually possible and must correct both the angulation of the ulna and the dislocated radial head. In instances in which the dislocation cannot be maintained in stable reduction, then open reduction of the radial head is necessary. After treatment, the elbow should be immobilized in flexion for a period of four to six weeks.

Fractures of the neck of the radius in

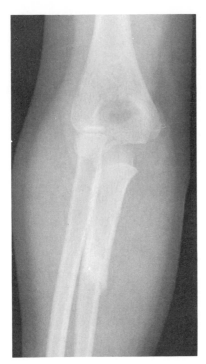

Figure 2–21. Monteggia's fracture of the right forearm. Note the overriding of the ulna and the dislocation of the radial head. Soft tissue swelling is also evident.

children occur from falls onto the outstretched upper extremity (Fig. 2–22). Treatment depends upon the degree of angulation of the radial neck. Angulation of less than 10 to 15 degrees requires only immobilization for three weeks. Angulation of greater than 15 to 20 degrees should be treated by closed or, if not possible, open reduction in order to prevent loss of forearm rotation after malunion.

THE ELBOW

Congenital Dislocation

Total congenital dislocation of the radius and ulna at the elbow is very uncommon as an isolated event and is most often associated with multiple dislocations in entities such as Larsen's syndrome.

More common is congenital dislocation of the head of the radius (Fig. 2–23). This may occur in isolation or may be associated with other conditions such as radioulnar synostosis, Larsen's syndrome, and arthrogryposis multiplex congenita. Since function is usually quite good, even with complete dislocation, this condition is usually not detected in the neonatal or even in the infantile period. The radial head is dislocated laterally and posteriorly, and overgrowth results, presenting as

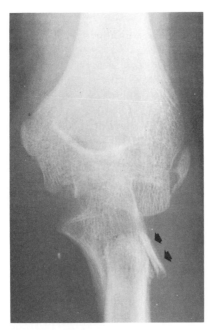

Figure 2–22. AP view of the left elbow demonstrating a markedly displaced fracture of the hand and neck of the radius.

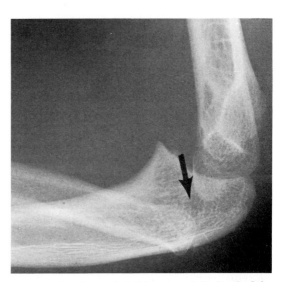

Figure 2–23. Congenital dislocation of the head of the radius. Note that the radial shaft does not point at the humeral capitellum.

a posterior-lateral prominence at the elbow. Some limitation of supination is usually present. Often, the condition is first noticed after an injury to the upper extremity, and it then could be mistaken for an acute dislocation. In this regard, comparison views of both forearms in their entirety are invaluable. Congenital dislocation of the radial head should not be treated. Attempts at open reduction universally fail, and excision of the radial head in a child usually will result in growth deformities of the forearm and wrist.

Although congenital anterior dislocation of the radial head can occur, it also results in minimal functional impairment and requires no treatment.

Little League Elbow

Little League elbow is an overuse syndrome occurring most commonly in young baseball pitchers between the ages of nine and 13 years. Symptoms are based on the fact that throwing produces markedly increased tension or distraction forces on the medial side of the elbow and strong compressive forces on the lateral or radial-capitellar side. There may be hypertrophy of the ulna or of the distal humerus. Because of this, pain and swelling may be seen on the medial, the lateral, or the posterior aspect of the elbow region, the latter occurring when the hypertrophic olecranon process of the ulna impinges upon the olecranon fossa of the humerus.

The common injury seen on the medial side of the elbow is strain or separation of the medial epicondyle with fragmentation or calcification in the adjacent soft tissues. On the posterior aspect, calcification of the olecranon fossa and elongation of the olecranon are often noted. On the lateral side, compressive injuries to the capitellum produce sclerosis and irregularity mimicking osteochondral fractures or Panner's disease, or both. Occasionally, angulated deformities of the radial head and neck are also seen.

Statistically, medial side injuries are more common than those on the lateral side and respond to cessation of the overloading activity. The best treatment, then, is prevention. This involves education of the players, the parents, and the coaches, which is sometimes quite difficult. Power-building exercises and avoidance of throwing "breaking pitches" or "curve balls" in the junior baseball leagues

are wise. Perhaps the best advice is to note that little leaguers with elbow pain make excellent first basemen.

Nursemaid's Elbow ("Pulled" Elbow)

This is a common injury in the preschool-aged child. It is produced by sudden jerking, with longitudinal and pronation force, when the child is grabbed by the forearm or wrist. The injury commonly occurs in grocery stores, on stairways or steps, or in other situations when the parent, sibling, or attendant is in a hurry or the child is misbehaving. The child presents with a painful flexed and pronated elbow which he clamps to his side and refuses to allow anyone to touch.

The injury is produced by a sudden tearing of the annular ligament surrounding the radial neck. It is a transient subluxation wherein the radial head temporarily loses continuity with the capitellum. In the interval, the proximal portion of the ligament becomes impaled between the joint surfaces when the traction is released. Because of this, radiographic examination always shows normal findings, the trapped ligament being radiolucent.

The most universally successful treatment consists of quick supination of the forearm with the elbow in flexion. This is not infrequently accomplished by the radiographic technician, who unknowingly cures the lesion while attempting to position the elbow for an anteroposterior (AP) view. Shortly after release of the ligament, the pain disappears, and the child begins to use the arm in a normal fashion. It is good to add a posterior splint for a period of 10 to 14 days to allow for healing of the partially torn ligament. Treatment is completed by educating the parents, babysitters, and siblings about the disorder and about the necessity to avoid this type of modification of misbehavior.

Panner's Disease

Panner's disease is avascular necrosis of the capitellum of the humerus. The afflicted child presents with pain and occasionally mild swelling around the elbow. There may be some loss of motion as well. The condition occurs most often in mid or late childhood.

The diagnosis is made by radiographic examination, which usually shows sclerosis,

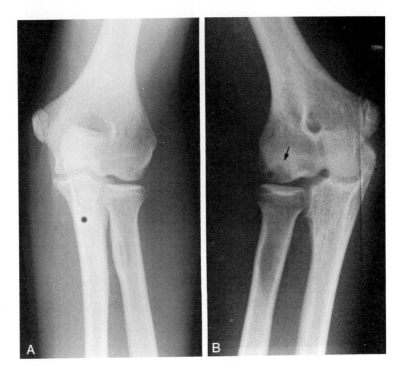

Figure 2–24. *A,* Normal left elbow of a 13-year-old girl. *B,* Right elbow of the same girl. Note the lytic defect in the capitellum of the humerus. This represents very early Panner's disease. The lesion healed without treatment.

irregularity, and loss of height of the capitellum. Comparison views are helpful in mild cases (Fig. 2–24). This lesion is best managed by symptomatic treatment, including mild analgesics, self-restriction of activities, and perhaps a sling or posterior splint when the disorder is most symptomatic. Panner's disease is usually self-limited and most often does not result in deformity or early degenerative arthritis.

Osteochondral Fracture of the Capitellum

This is an acute traumatic lesion that may give the appearance of Panner's disease but is differentiated from it by a history of acute trauma, usually a fall onto the outstretched upper limb. The radius compresses the capitellum and causes either a compression or a chip fracture. Compression fractures are best treated with use of a sling until the swelling and pain are resolved. Then early active motion of the elbow can begin. A chip fracture, if trapped in the joint or of sufficient magnitude to interfere with the articular surface, should be treated with open reduction and internal fixation. Excision of small chips is permissible.

Traumatic Dislocation of the Elbow

Dislocation of both the radius and the ulna at the elbow joint is an unusual injury in children, occurring mostly in adolescents and adults. Although it is possible to have a true dislocation in a younger child, this is extremely rare and usually represents fracture through the distal humerus, much of which is cartilaginous in early childhood. In diagnosing traumatic lesions around the elbow in children, it is essential to compare radiographs of the affected side with some of the normal side.

When dislocation does occur, it is often accompanied by fracture of the proximal ulna, radial neck, or one of the humeral epicondyles (Fig. 2–25). Substantial force is required to produce this injury, and one should always look for neurovascular disruption and a possible forearm compartment syndrome.

The treatment of traumatic elbow dislocation consists of closed reduction performed with the patient under adequate anesthesia. Following reduction, the elbow should be immobilized at 90 degrees of flexion for two to three weeks to allow soft tissue healing to occur. Permanent loss of some motion is the rule.

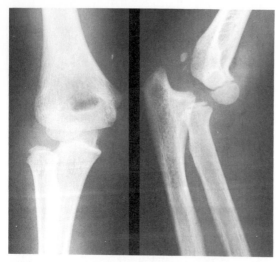

Figure 2–25. AP and slightly oblique lateral view of the right elbow, showing dislocation. Note that the head of the radius is no longer in a normal articular relationship with the humeral capitellum. The medial humeral epicondyle is beginning to ossify. There is a small avulsion fragment from the distal humerus.

FRACTURES OF THE DISTAL HUMERUS

The most common distal humeral fractures in children are lateral condylar, medial epi-condylar, transphyseal, and supracondylar fractures.

Lateral Condylar Fractures

These common fractures are usually caused by a shearing off of the capitellum by the compressive force of the radius during a fall onto the outstretched arm (Fig. 2–26). The fracture is intra-articular and disrupts the joint surface, crosses through the epiphysis, traverses the growth plate, and extends further proximally, disrupting the lateral cortex of the humeral metaphysis.

Lateral condylar fractures have great potential for resulting in deformity and interfering with function unless open reduction, with anatomic reapproximation of the fragments and internal fixation, is carried out. If anatomic reduction is not achieved, bony union across the growth plate will occur, and progressive angular deformity will be the result. This is cosmetically displeasing and may produce a traction neuropraxia of the ulnar nerve. The vast majority, if not all, of these acute fractures require open treatment. If one opts for closed treatment of a nondisplaced fracture, extremely close follow-up is necessary because these fractures are noto-

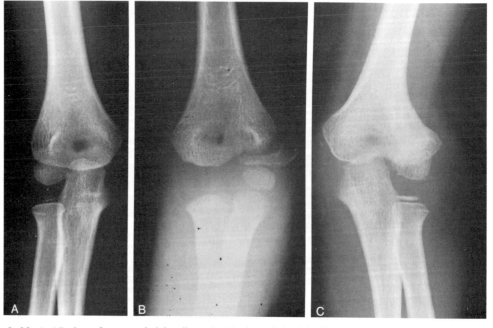

Figure 2–26. *A*, AP view of a normal right elbow. *B*, AP view of the left elbow, showing a displaced fracture of the lateral humeral condyle. This fracture was not treated with appropriate open reduction. *C*, Eighteen months later, there are early signs of deformity with valgus angulation at the elbow.

riously unstable and may become displaced, even in an appropriate cast.

Medial Epicondylar Fractures

These are avulsion injuries usually resulting from an angular stress on the extended elbow or occurring concomitantly with dislocation of the elbow (Fig. 2–27). Most will do well with immobilization alone, and no specific attempt at reduction is necessary. Most heal by strong fibrous union without resultant functional or cosmetic deficit. Only if the elbow is grossly unstable or the fracture fragment is large and rotated or trapped within the elbow joint is open reduction necessary. Because of the angular force required to produce this fracture, one should carefully evaluate the neurologic status of the arm, particularly of the ulnar nerve.

Transphyseal Fractures

These injuries are fracture-separations through the distal humeral physis, and they usually occur in infants and young children (Fig. 2–28). The cause is most often a sudden longitudinal jerk or a rotatory shearing force. For this reason, they are frequently associ-

ated with child abuse. The diagnosis is suspected by detecting the massive swelling around the elbow that always accompanies this fracture. Although most of the distal humerus is cartilaginous in young children, comparison radiographs of the affected and the normal elbows will almost always show posteromedial displacement of the distal fragment. Treatment consists of closed reduction followed by immobilization for three weeks with the elbow in flexion and pronation.

Supracondylar Fractures

These lesions are especially significant and especially common in active children. Most often, they are the result of hyperextension of the elbow, although they may be produced by direct axial force along the forearm with the elbow flexed. When one considers that the ulna wraps around the distal humerus like a wrench around a nut, it is easy to see how this transverse fracture above the level of the humeral condyles can occur. There is usually posterior displacement of the distal fragment (Fig. 2–29).

Of particular concern with this injury is the potential for disruption of blood supply to the forearm and hand due to laceration

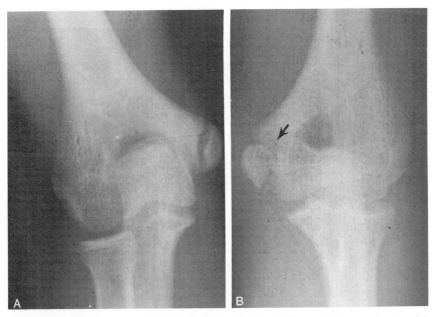

Figure 2–27. *A,* AP view of a normal right elbow. Note the anatomy of the medial humeral epicondyle. *B,* Fracture of the medial epicondyle of the left humerus. Note rotation of the epicondylar fracture fragment.

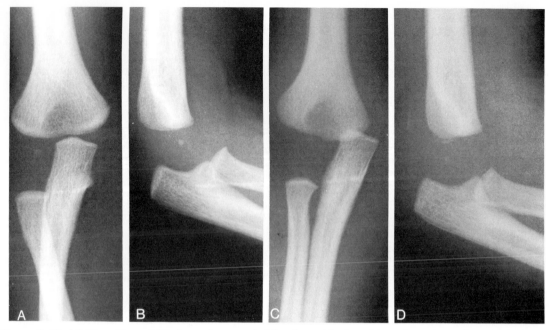

Figure 2–28. AP *(A)* and lateral *(B)* views of a normal right elbow, AP *(C)* and lateral *(D)* views of a posteriorly and medially displaced fracture through the distal humeral growth plate. A small metaphyseal fracture fragment is visible on the lateral view.

or compression of the major arteries crossing the elbow. This can result in Volkmann's ischemic contracture and paralysis, a catastrophic injury.

A supracondylar fracture is a true orthopedic emergency and demands immediate treatment of the highest proficiency. The most important aspect of treatment is to preserve the vascular and neurologic function in the extremity. Undisplaced fractures are treated with immobilization in a position of flexion for a period of three to six weeks. Displaced fractures may be treated with closed reduction, skeletal traction, or open

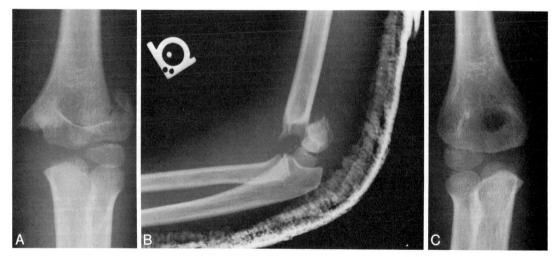

Figure 2–29. AP *(A)* and lateral *(B)* views of a posteriorly and laterally displaced supracondylar fracture of the distal humerus. *C,* The normal elbow for comparison.

reduction and internal fixation, depending upon the individual case. These are difficult fractures to treat, and compulsive care is necessary if malunion and subsequent angulation are to be prevented. In some cases, these are simply unavoidable, and a corrective osteotomy may be necessary at an older age.

THE HUMERUS

Unicameral Bone Cyst

A unicameral bone cyst is a benign cavitary lesion often occurring in the metaphyseal region of the proximal humerus, either adjacent to (active cyst) or a short distance away from (passive cyst) the growth plate (Fig. 2–30). These lesions are usually first detected because of their presentation as a pathologic fracture. The principle of management is to prevent recurrent fractures. In the past, the treatment of choice has been to allow healing of the acute disorder followed by elective curettage, with or without bone grafting, to entice the cyst to fill in and heal. Presently, intralesional injections of steroids have been

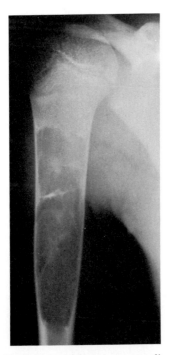

Figure 2–30. Unicameral bone cyst not adjacent to the growth plate in the right humerus.

reasonably successful, although repeat injections may be necessary.

Fracture of the Shaft of the Humerus

This is not a common injury in children, but when it occurs, it may be associated with a transient radial nerve palsy. Depending upon the amount of force that produced the fracture, the trauma to the nerve may take several weeks to several months to resolve. The type of immobilization following closed reduction depends upon the stability of the fracture and can range from use of a sling and swathe (Velpeau) bandage to use of a formal shoulder spica cast. Closed treatment is almost always successful with humeral shaft fractures in children.

Fractures of the Proximal Humerus

Bony injuries to the proximal humerus most often occur just before or throughout the adolescent growth spurt. The fracture usually involves the growth plate and may be a complete epiphyseal separation or may have a small metaphyseal fragment attached. The injury is easily diagnosed from study of AP and axillary view radiographs, which may show minimal or substantial displacement. For mild displacement, reduction is frequently unnecessary, and immobilization of the shoulder in a sling and swathe for a period of three to six weeks, depending upon the age of the patient, is usually adequate. The more displaced fractures are best treated with closed reduction. Open reduction and intramedullary fixation are rarely necessary.

THE SHOULDER

Sprengel's Deformity

The scapula develops in the cervical region and normally descends during fetal life. Sprengel's deformity is a failure of descent of the scapula and may be unilateral or, in one third of cases, bilateral. It is characterized by a somewhat hypoplastic and malrotated scapula, which is often fixed to the posterior cervical spinous processes by either a bony connection (omovertebral bone) or a fibrous or fibrocartilaginous band (Fig. 2–31). There is some limitation of shoulder abduction and,

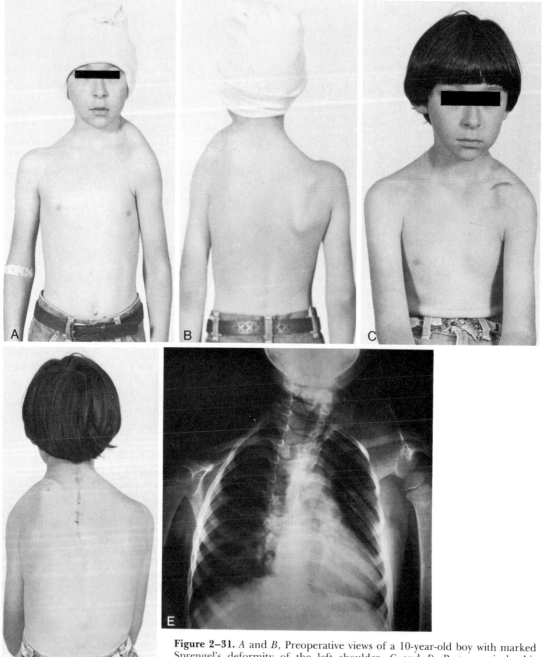

Figure 2–31. *A* and *B*, Preoperative views of a 10-year-old boy with marked Sprengel's deformity of the left shoulder. *C* and *D*, Postoperatively, his appearance is improved, although there was little gain in motion. *E*, Radiograph of the same patient's left Sprengel's deformity. Note the rotation and congenital elevation of the left scapula. The omovertebral bone can be seen extending from the cervical spine toward the scapula.

to a lesser extent, of forward flexion, both of which are secondary to malrotation and restriction of scapular-thoracic motion. Unless the condition is bilateral, function is usually quite good, and treatment is indicated for cosmetic reasons only. It is essential to note that abnormalities such as congenital spinal problems and renal anomalies are frequently associated with Sprengel's deformity.

Treatment requires surgical release of the scapula and its proximal omovertebral tether and usually includes osteotomy or morselization of the clavicle, resection of the supraspinous portion of the scapula, and muscle transfers. This is a procedure of major magnitude that produces a substantial scar and should be done only for severe cases.

Absence of the Pectoral Musculature

The pectoralis major is the most commonly absent muscle in the body. When it is absent, one must look for other anomalies such as syndactyly and cardiac lesions. Although absence of the pectoral musculature may present a mild to moderate cosmetic deformity, function is usually normal, and treatment is unnecessary.

Erb's Palsy ("Obstetric Paralysis")

Erb's palsy results from stretching injuries to the components of the brachial plexus incurred during delivery and is seen most often following the difficult deliveries of large babies. It is good to tell the parents that although the injury is probably related to the obstetric procedure, the alternative to prompt intervention at the appropriate time would most likely have been a severe cerebral insult or even death. The spectrum of injuries to the brachial plexus extends from a transient mild stretching to complete disruption of the continuity of the nerve trunks, cords, or nerve roots. The lesion produced is a lower motor neuron or flaccid one, with sensory involvement in the more severe cases (Fig. 2–32). Three types of Erb's palsy have been described, based upon the anatomic level of the lesion. These are: (1) true Erb's palsy with involvement of the C5 and C6 nerve root distributions; (2) Erb-Duchenne-Klumpke palsy, wherein the entire brachial plexus from C4 or C5 to T1 is involved; and (3) Klumpke's palsy, in which the C8 and T1

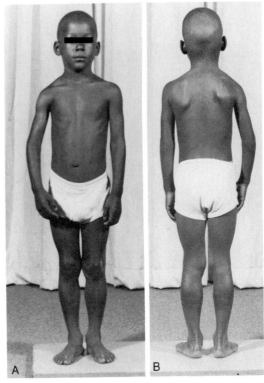

Figure 2–32. *A* and *B*, This patient has Erb's palsy of the right upper extremity. Note atrophy of the shoulder musculature, winging of the right scapula, and internal rotation at the shoulder.

nerve root distributions are involved. The Erb's type is more common than the other two types. In Erb's palsy, the deltoid and other shoulder muscles, as well as the biceps and brachioradialis muscles, are paretic. In the Erb-Duchenne-Klumpke type, which has the worst prognosis, the entire arm is flail. In the Klumpke type, the wrist and hand muscles are involved, with sparing of the shoulder girdle and elbow flexors. Horner's syndrome is often seen with the Klumpke type.

The diagnosis is established by careful motor examination of the infant. In the neonatal period, fracture of the humerus or clavicle, or fracture or dislocation of the cervical spine, should be ruled out by use of plain radiographic examination or tomography. Myelography and electrodiagnostic studies are sometimes necessary.

The natural course of brachial plexus palsy depends on the disease. If complete disruption has occurred, there will be no return of neurologic function. Although primary surgical repair of the involved neurologic struc-

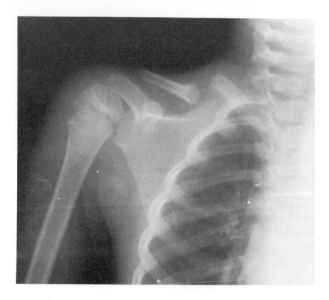

Figure 2–33. Congenital pseudarthrosis of the right clavicle. Note the caudal displacement of the lateral clavicular segment secondary to the weight of the upper limb.

tures appears attractive, this technique has not had wide application or success.

In cases in which the nerve trunks are not disrupted, return of neurologic function is very possible. While most children will not fully recover, many do gain significant functional improvement, particularly within the first year of life. For this reason, the initial treatment should be based on the premise that some neurologic recovery may occur, and therefore daily range-of-motion exercises and removable splints may be quite helpful. If a significant neurologic deficit persists beyond the age of six years, and if the patient is cooperative, reconstructive surgical procedures and tendon transfers may be considered.

Congenital Pseudarthrosis of the Clavicle

This condition may mimic a fracture of the clavicle developed at or shortly after birth. No amount of immobilization, however, will induce healing to occur. The cause is unknown. The patient presents with a defect in the central third of the clavicle, noted on clinical examination as a painless lump (Fig. 2–33). In most cases, some degree of motion between the bony ends is detectable. The condition is far more common the right side than on the left. The shoulder on the involved side may that on appear lower than that on the uninvolved side and may be rotated slightly forward. Weakness and loss of function are transient and rarely seen.

Treatment is not indicated unless the cosmetic deformity merits trading a lump for a scar. The development of pain is extremely uncommon in this condition but is the major indication for surgical correction, which consists of internal fixation and bone grafting. Congenital pseudarthrosis should be differentiated from variants of cleidocranial dysostosis and neurofibromatosis.

Fracture of the Clavicle

This is a common injury throughout childhood, from birth through maturity (Fig. 2–34). Younger children are more apt to have incomplete fractures, whereas complete fractures of the middle third of the clavicle are the rule in the older children. The diagnosis is not difficult: The patient presents with a history of trauma and a painful lump, often with crepitation, over the fracture site. Neurovascular complications are much less common than one might expect, given the proximity of the underlying brachial plexus, apex of the lung, and subclavian artery and vein.

The treatment of a fractured clavicle is relatively simple, and nonunion is extremely uncommon. Appropriate treatment consists of use of a soft, padded, figure-eight clavicle strap to hold the shoulder up and back. A sling may also be useful in this regard, as well as in increasing the child's comfort. The "immobilization" does not completely prevent motion at the fracture site, and, there

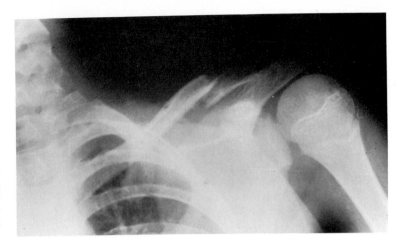

Figure 2–34. Transverse fracture of the distal left clavicle with overriding. Such fractures heal promptly with three weeks of immobilization in a figure-of-eight splint.

fore, these lesions heal with a large firm callus, which is readily seen and felt. Reassurance to the parents that this will remodel completely within a year's time is wise.

Dislocation of the Shoulder

Dislocation of the shoulder joint is extremely rare in young children. It becomes more common in adolescents and is seen most often in young adults (Fig. 2–35). Because the glenoid fossa, with which the humeral head articulates, faces slightly anteriorly, the usual position of dislocation is with the humeral head displaced anteriorly and inferiorly beneath the coracoid process of the scapula. This is the so-called "anterior" or "subcoracoid" dislocation. Less common are the true posterior dislocations, caused by a direct force applied to the anterior surface of the shoulder or by a fall onto the outstretched upper extremity. Even less common are the inferior dislocations, which present with the arm in a position of full abduction, the "luxatio erecta" postion. Any dislocation may produce stretching of the neurologic components of the brachial plexus, although this is actually quite rare. More commonly seen is an area of hypesthesia over the deltoid, caused by neuropraxia of the axillary nerve.

Confirmation of dislocation of the shoulder

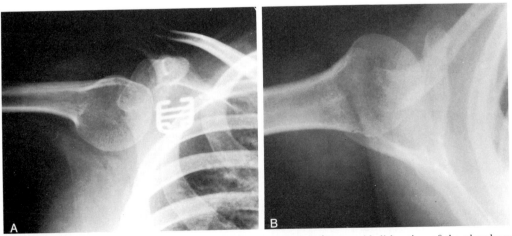

Figure 2–35. *A,* AP view of the right shoulder showing an anterior subcoracoid dislocation of the glenohumeral joint. Note that the humeral head is displaced inferiorly and medially to the glenoid. *B,* An axillary view (looking up) taken at 90 degrees to the AP plane shows the anterior displacement of the humeral head.

is best done by obtaining an AP and a true axillary radiographic view, both easily obtainable without moving the shoulder. Closed reduction should be done by gentle means, and there are a variety of standard ways of accomplishing this, depending upon the position of dislocation. All initial dislocations and most second dislocations should be immobilized three to six weeks to allow for healing of the torn and stretched soft tissue structures. Even so, recurrent dislocation of the shoulder is common in active young people. Following the second or third dislocation, further recurrences are the rule, and it is wise to consider surgical repair.

Habitual or voluntary dislocation of the shoulder is occasionally seen in young children and adolescents. Usually, there is no antecedent history of trauma, and the voluntary dislocation or subluxation is painless. The best approach to this situation is carefully to counsel the patient and the parents that there is a risk of pain and arthritis in the long run if such behavior continues. A high incidence of emotional and behavioral disorders accompanies this phenomenon and makes psychologic counseling the treatment of choice in many cases. Surgical results in voluntary dislocation of the shoulder are almost uniformly dismal.

Some children, particularly those with increased ligamentous laxity, are plagued by recurrent involuntary subluxation of the shoulder. Many can eventually reproduce the subluxation voluntarily. While muscle strengthening exercises may be prescribed, the best treatment is reassurance and advising the child not to do this voluntarily. Surgical results in recurrent mild subluxation are not very good.

References

Syndactyly

Ruby L and Goldberg MJ: Syndactyly and polydactyly. Orthop Clin North Am 7:361, 1976.
Toledo LC and Ger E: Evaluation of the operative treatment of syndactyly. J Hand Surg 4:556, 1979.

Polydactyly

Miura T: Duplicated thumb. J Plast Reconstr Surg 69:470, 1982.
Wood VE: Polydactyly and the triphalangeal thumb. J Hand Surg 3:436, 1978.

Macrodactyly

Barsky AJ: Mactodactyly. J Bone Joint Surg 49A:1255, 1967.

Rechnagel K: Megalodactylism. Report of 7 cases. Acta Orthop Scand 38:57, 1967.

Clinodactyly and Kirner's Deformity

Burke F and Flatt A: Clinodactyly. A review of a series of cases. Hand 11:269, 1979.
Carstam N and Eiken O: Kirner's deformity of the little finger. Case reports and proposed treatment. J Bone Joint Surg 52A:1663, 1970.
Dykes RG: Kirner's deformity of the little finger. J Bone Joint Surg 60B:58, 1978.
Poznanski, AK et al.: Clinodactyly, camptodactyly, Kirner's deformity, and other crooked fingers. Radiology 93:573, 1969.

Camptodactyly

Smith RJ and Kaplan EB: Camptodactyly and similar atraumatic flexion deformities of the proximal interphalangeal joints of the fingers. J Bone Joint Surg 50A:1187, 1968.

Ectrodactyly

Barsky AJ: Cleft hand. Classification, incidence, and treatment: Review of the literature and report of nineteen cases. J Bone Joint Surg 46:1707, 1964.
Nutt JN III and Flatt A: Congenital central hand deficit. J Hand Surg 6:48, 1981.

Symphalangism

Flatt AE and Wood VE: Rigid digits or symphalangism. Hand 7:197, 1975.
Geelhoed GW et al.: Symphalangism and tarsal coalitions: A hereditary syndrome. A report on two families. J Bone Joint Surg 51B:278, 1969.
Strasburger AK et al.: Symphalangism: Genetic and clinical aspects. Bull Johns Hopkins Hosp 117:108, 1965.

Trigger Thumb

Dinham JM and Meggitt BF: Trigger thumbs in children. J Bone Joint Surg 56B:153, 1974.
Weckesser EC et al.: Congenital clasp thumb (congenital flexion-adduction deformity of the thumb). J Bone Joint Surg 50A:1417, 1968.

Triphalangeal Thumb

Poznanski AK et al.: The thumb in congenital malformation syndromes. Radiology 100:115, 1971.

Hand Fractures and Dislocations

Barton J: Fractures of the phalanges of the hand in children. Hand 11:134, 1979.
Das SK and Brown HG: Management of lost fingertips in children. Hand 10:16, 1978.
Leonard MH and Dubravcik P: Management of fractured fingers in the child. Clin Orthop 73:160, 1970.
Rosenthal LJ et al.: Nonoperative management of distal fingertip amputation in children. Pediatrics 64:1, 1979.

Congenital Deficiency of the Radius

Bora FW Jr et al.: Radial meromelia. The deformity and its treatment. J Bone Joint Surg 52A:966, 1970.

Carroll RE and Louis DS: Anomalies associated with radial dysplasia. J Pediatr 84:409, 1974.

Gilbert A: Toe transfers for congenital hand defects. J Hand Surg 7:118, 1982.

Goldberg NH and Watson HK: Composite toe (phalanx and epiphysis) transfers in the reconstruction of the aphalangic hand. J Hand Surg 7:454, 1982.

Lamb DW: Radial club hand. A continuing study of 68 patients with 117 club hands. J Bone Joint Surg 59A:1, 1977.

Manske PR et al.: Centralization of the radial club hand: An ulnar surgical approach. J Hand Surg 6:423, 1981.

Quan L and Smith DW: The VATER Association: Vertebral defects; anal atresia, TE fistula and esophageal atresia, radial and renal dysplasia: a spectrum of associated defects. J Pediatr 82:104, 1973.

Roberts J et al.: Congenital absence of the radius. South Med J 73:702, 1980.

Shaperman J and Sumida CT: Recent advances in research and prosthetics for children. Clin Orthop 148:26, 1980.

Swanson AB: A classification for congenital limb malformations. J Hand Surg 1:8, 1976.

Congenital Deficiency of the Ulna

Blair WF et al.: Functional status in ulnar deficiency. J Pediatr Orthop 3:37, 1983.

Broudy AS and Smith RJ: Deformities of the hand and wrist with ulnar deficiency. J Hand Surg 4:304, 1979.

Ogden JA et al.: Ulnar dysmelia. J Bone Joint Surg 50A:467, 1978.

Straub LR: Congenital absence of the ulna. Am J Surg 109:1300, 1965.

Congenital Band Syndrome

Field JH and Krag DO: Congenital constricting bands and congenital amputation of the fingers: Placental studies. J Bone Joint Surg 55A:1035, 1973.

Izumi AK and Arnold HL Jr: Congenital annular bands (pseudoainhum) associated with other congenital anomalies. J Am Med Assoc 229:1208, 1974.

Kino Y: Clinical and experimental studies of the congenital constriction band syndrome with an emphasis on its etiology. J Bone Joint Surg 57A:636, 1975.

Moses JM et al.: Annular constricting bands. J Bone Joint Surg 61A:562, 1979.

Radioulnar Synostosis

Green WT and Mital MA: Congenital radioulnar synostosis: Surgical treatment. J Bone Joint Surg 61A:738, 1979.

Hansen OH and Andersen NO: Congenital radioulnar synostosis. A report of thirty-seven cases. Acta Orthop Scand 41:25, 1970.

Jancu J: Radio-ulnar synostosis: A common occurrence in sex chromosomal abnormalities. Am J Dis Child 122:10, 1971.

Mital MA: Congenital radioulnar synostosis and congenital dislocation of the radial head. Orthop Clin North Amer 7:375, 1976.

Madelung's Deformity

Dawe C et al.: Clinical variation in dyschondrosteosis: A report on thirteen individuals in eight families. J Bone Joint Surg 64B:377, 1982.

Golding JSR and Blackburne JS: Madelung's disease of the wrist and dyschondrosteosis. J Bone Joint Surg 58B:350, 1976.

Wrist Fractures

Rang, M: Children's Fractures. Philadelphia, JB Lippincott Co, 1974.

Salter RB and Harris WR: Injuries involving the epiphyseal plate. J Bone Joint Surg 45A:587, 1963.

Vahvanen V and Westerlund M: Fracture of the carpal scaphoid in children: A clinical and roentgenological study of 108 cases. Acta Orthop Scand 51:909, 1980.

Forearm Fractures

Blount WP: Fractures in Children. Baltimore, Williams and Wilkins, 1955.

Daruwalla JS: A study of radio-ulnar movements following fractures of the forearm in children. Clin Orthop 139:114, 1979.

Davis DR and Green DP: Forearm fractures in children. Clin Orthop 120:172, 1976.

Fuller DJ and McCullough CJ: Malunited fractures of the forearm in children. J Bone Joint Surg 64B;364, 1982.

Gelberman RA et al.: Compartment syndromes of the forearm: Diagnosis and treatment. Clin Orthop 161:252, 1981.

Piero A et al.: Acute Monteggia lesions in children. J Bone Joint Surg 59A:92, 1977.

Tibone JE and Stoltz M: Fractures of the radial head and neck in children. J Bone Joint Surg 63A:100, 1981.

Silberstein MJ et al.: Some vagaries of the radial head and neck. J Bone Joint Surg 64A:1153, 1982.

Congenital Dislocation of the Elbow and Radial Head

Almquist EE et al.: Congenital dislocation of the head of the radius. J Bone Surg 51A:1118, 1969.

Caravias DE: Some observations on congenital dislocation of the head of the radius. J Bone Joint Surg 39B:860, 1957.

Kelly DW: Congenital dislocation of the radial head: Spectrum and natural history. J Pediatr Orthop 1:295, 1981.

Lloyd-Roberts GC and Bucknill TM: Anterior dislocation of the radial head in children. J Bone Joint Surg 59B:402, 1977.

Little League Elbow

Pappas AM; Elbow problems associated with baseball during childhood and adolescence. Clin Orthop 164:30, 1982.

Nursemaid's Elbow

Ryan JR: The relationship of the radial head to radial neck diameters in fetuses and adults with reference to radial head subluxation in children. J Bone Joint Surg 51A:781, 1969.

Salter RB and Zaltz C: Anatomic investigations of the mechanism of injury and pathologic anatomy of pulled elbow in young children. Clin Orthop 77:134, 1971.

Panner's Disease

Smith MGH: Osteochondritis of the humeral capitellum. J Bone Joint Surg 46B:50, 1964.

Woodward AH and Bianco AJ Jr: Osteochondritis dissecans of the elbow. Clin Orthop 110:35, 1975.

Traumatic Dislocation of the Elbow

Carlioz H and Abols Y: Posterior dislocation of the elbow in children. J Pediatr Orthop 4:8, 1984.

Lateral Humeral Condylar Fractures

Fontanetta P et al.: Missed, maluniting, and malunited fractures of the lateral humeral condyle in children. J Trauma 18:329, 1978.

Silberstein MJ et al.: Some vagaries of the lateral epicondyle. J Bone Joint Surg 64A:444, 1982.

Medial Humeral Epicondylar Fractures

Fowles JV and Kassab MT: Displaced fractures of the medial humeral condyle in children. J Bone Joint Surg 62A:1159, 1980.

Silberstein MJ et al: Some vagaries of the medial epicondyle. J Bone Joint Surg 63A:524, 1981.

Transphyseal Humeral Fractures

DeLee JC et al.: Fracture-separation of the distal humeral epiphysis. J Bone Joint Surg 62A:46, 1980.

Supracondylar Humeral Fractures

Arino VL et al.: Percutaneous fixation of supracondylar fractures of the humerus in children. J Bone Joint Surg 59A:914, 1977.

Buhl O and Hellberg S: Displaced supracondylar fractures of the humerus in children. Acta Orthop Scand 53:67, 1982.

Dameron TB Jr: Transverse fractures of the distal humerus in children. American Academy of Orthopaedic Surgeons Instructional Course Lectures, 30:224. St. Louis, CV Mosby Co, 1981.

Labelle H et al.: Cubitus varus deformity following supracondylar fractures of the humerus in children. J Pediatr Orthop 2:539, 1982.

Prietto CA: Supracondylar fractures of the humerus. J Bone Joint Surg 61A:425, 1979.

Smith L: Deformity following supracondylar fracture of the humerus. J Bone Joint Surg 42A:235, 1960.

Unicameral Bone Cyst

Oppenheim WL and Galleno H: Operative treatment versus steroid injection in the management of unicameral bone cysts. J Pediatr Orthop 4:1, 1984.

Fracture of the Shaft and Proximal Humerus

Campbell J and Almand HGA: Fracture separation of the proximal humeral epiphysis. J Bone Joint Surg 59A:262, 1977.

Kohler RN and Trillaud JM: Fracture and fracture separation of the proximal humerus in children: Report of 136 cases. J Pediatr Orthop 3:326, 1983.

Sprengel's Deformity

Carson WG et al.: Congenital elevation of the scapula.

Surgical correction by the Woodward procedure. J Bone Joint Surg 63A:1199, 1981.

Klisic P et al.: Relocation of congenitally elevated scapula. J Pediatr Orthop 1:43, 1981.

Woodward JW: Congenital elevation of the scapula. Correction by release and transplantation of muscle origins. J Bone Joint Surg 43A:219, 1961.

Absence of the Pectoral Musculature

Renshaw TS: Congenital Muscular Defects. *In* Gellis SS and Kagan BM (eds): Current Pediatric Therapy, 11th ed, p 413. Philadelphia, WB Saunders Co, 1984.

Resnick E: Congenital unilateral absence of the pectoral muscles often associated with syndactylism. J Bone Joint Surg 24:925, 1942.

Erb's Palsy

Adler JB and Patterson RL Jr: Erb's palsy: Long-term results of therapy in 88 cases. J Bone Joint Surg 49A:1052, 1967.

Eng GD et al.: Brachial plexus palsy in neonates and children. Arch Phys Med Rehabil 59:458, 1978.

Hoffer M et al.: Functional recovery and orthopaedic management of brachial plexus palsies. J Am Med Assoc 246:2467, 1982.

Solonen KA et al.: Early reconstruction in the birth injuries of the brachial plexus. J Pediatr Orthop 1:367, 1981.

Tada K et al.: Birth palsy: Natural recovery course and combined root avulsion. J Pediatr Orthop 4:279, 1984.

Congenital Pseudarthrosis of the Clavicle

Ahmadi B and Steel HH: Congenital pseudarthrosis of the clavicle. Clin Orthop 126:130, 1977.

Gibson DA and Carroll N: Congenital pseudarthrosis of the clavicle. J Bone Joint Surg 52B:629, 1970.

Kohler R et al.: Congenital pseudarthrosis of the clavicle. A report of seven cases. Chir Pediatr 21:201, 1980.

Quinlan WR et al.: Congenital pseudarthrosis of the clavicle. Acta Orthop Scand 51:489, 1980.

Wall JJ: Congenital pseudarthrosis in the clavicle. J Bone Joint Surg 52A:1003, 1970.

Fracture of the Clavicle

Conwell HE: Fractures of the clavicle, simple fixation dressing with summary of treatment and results attained in 92 cases. J Am Med Assoc 90:838, 1928.

McCally WC and Kelly DA: Treatment of fractures of the clavicle, ribs, and scapulae. Am J Surg 50:558, 1940.

Dislocation of the Shoulder

Protzman RR: Anterior instability of the shoulder. J Bone Joint Surg 62A:909, 1980.

Rowe CR et al.: Voluntary dislocation of the shoulder. J Bone Joint Surg 55A:445, 1973.

Rowe CR and Zarins B: Recurrent transient subluxation of the shoulder. J Bone Joint Surg 63A:863, 1981.

Wagner KT and Lyne ED: Adolescent traumatic dislocations of the shoulder with open epiphyses. J Pediatr Orthop 3:61, 1983.

3

The Spine

Certain spinal problems have great potential for interfering with the health of infants and children. Congenital anomalies can produce an insidious neurologic deficit, which may be permanent. A progressive deformity may lead to asymmetric stress on the facet joints of the spine with subsequent early degenerative arthritis and back pain. Pulmonary and other visceral compression due to shortening and deformity of the trunk and thorax can produce restrictive lung disease and cor pulmonale. Progressive scoliotic and kyphotic deformities can result in severe cosmetic disfigurement.

Despite their importance, spinal conditions often are not very obvious and may easily be overlooked. It is an excellent idea to examine periodically for spinal deformity in patients of the pediatric age group.

CONGENITAL DEFORMITIES

Myelodysplasia

The term "myelodysplasia" means abnormal development of the vertebral column or spinal cord or both. This can range from something as benign and innocuous as spina bifida occulta to something as profound as an open myelomeningocele, the most complex neuromuscular deformity compatible with life.

Spina bifida occulta is the failure of the posterior laminae of a vertebra to fuse in the midline and form a complete bony arch (Fig. 3–1). The incidence of this minor anomaly is about 5%. It is most commonly found in the lumbosacral region but is also seen in the thoracolumbar or cervicothoracic areas. Multiple areas of spina bifida occulta can occur. The significance of this finding in the lumbosacral region is that it increases the risk of development of either an elongation or a fatigue fracture of the pars interarticularis (spondylolysis) and increases the risk of subsequent vertebral slipping (spondylolisthesis).

More significant failure of fusion of the posterior elements of the spine usually leads to some herniation of the intact meninges, a meningocele (Fig. 3–2). By definition, this condition contains no neural elements, and neurologic function is intact. Meningoceles may be associated with neoplasia, particularly fatty tumors known a lipomeningoceles. These can involve neurologic structures and can be extremely difficult management problems because of their aggressive growth. Anterior meningoceles, which can also occur, present as intrapelvic soft masses. The uncomplicated posterior meningocele is covered with intact skin. It may enlarge, become uncomfortable, and be subject to trauma. If so, surgical repair is appropriate.

An open myelomeningocele containing abnormal neurologic elements is obvious at birth. This deformity is often associated with the Arnold-Chiari malformation, subsequent hydrocephalus, and profound neurologic deficit with motor loss, diminished or absent sensation, and bowel and bladder paralysis. It is most often seen in the lower half of the spine but can occur in the cervical region. In myelomeningocele, deformities and contractures of the lower extremities are usually present. Scoliosis is common, being more likely the more cephalic the level of the lesion. Maximum management means sur-

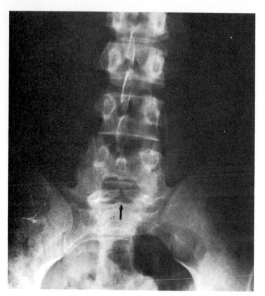

Figure 3–1. Spina bifida occulta of S1. Note that the laminae do not fuse in the midline.

gical closure of the defect, control of the hydrocephalus, and skilled nursing, pediatric, urologic, neurosurgical, and orthopedic care. These children should be managed by teams of interested specialists experienced in the treatment of myelomeningocele. This lesion is discussed in more detail in Chapter 7.

Diastematomyelia

In this condition, a stem or spike of bone, cartilage, fibrous tissue, or combinations of these tissues exist in the midline of the spinal canal in the anteroposterior plane. The lesion splits the spinal cord or nerve roots into two columns (diplomyelia) (Fig. 3–3). Diastematomyelia, while usually found in the thoracolumbar or lumbar region, may occur as a single phenomenon or at multiple levels. Cutaneous abnormalities over the lesion are often seen, the most common being either a dermal sinus or an area of hypertrichosis (Fig. 3–4).

The clinical significance of diastematomyelia is its potential effect as a tether stopping the normal proximal migration of the growing spinal cord, since the vertebral column normally lengthens at a faster rate than the spinal cord. Progressive neurologic deficit caused by a tethered spinal cord most often leads to lower extremity deformities, particularly of the foot and ankle; muscle weak-

ness; atrophy; and interference with bowel or bladder sphincter function. Other abnormalities such as Sprengel's deformity, congenital scoliosis, and urologic anomalies are commonly associated with diastematomyelia.

The diagnosis is suspected from the clinical findings and is confirmed by radiographic studies. Often, the midline bony mass may be identified on plain radiographs, although the most common findings are localized widening of the interpendicular distance and localized spina bifida occulta. The diagnosis is confirmed by ultrasonographic examination or by computerized tomographic scanning, usually augmented by myelography, since more than one stem or other intraspinal anomaly may be present.

In the past, prophylactic removal of these lesions was advocated by some, but currently the majority of neurosurgeons feel that this is not justified. The recommended treatment is careful periodic follow-up to document the absence of abnormal neurologic findings. The presence of a diastematomyelia does not automatically imply tethering of the spinal cord.

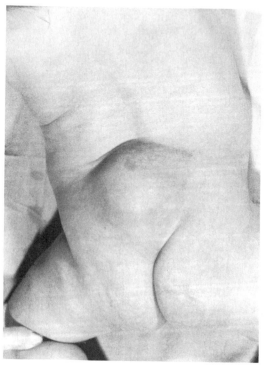

Figure 3–2. A closed meningocele with slight hyperpigmentation in an infant who had completely normal neurologic function but had congenital scoliosis.

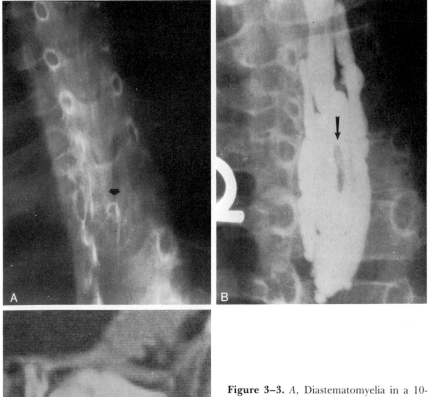

Figure 3–3. *A,* Diastematomyelia in a 10-year-old boy. Note the spike of bone in the center of the vertebral canal and the widening of the interpedicular distance at the level of the lesion. *B,* Myelogram of a patient with diastematomyelia. Note the passage of dye around the lesion and the widening of the spinal canal. *C,* Diastematomyelia as shown by computerized tomography. Note the bony spike dividing the spinal canal into two compartments and splitting the spinal cord.

Cervical Spine Problems

Developmental conditions of the cervical spine are frequently associated with torticollis or neurologic problems. Several well-defined anomalies can occur in this region.

Laxity of the transverse atlantal ligament may be congenital or may result from trauma or from inflammatory conditions such as nearby pharyngeal infections or juvenile rheumatoid arthritis. It is sometimes associated with odontoid hypoplasia in Morquio's disease or in spondyloepiphyseal dysplasia. It also occurs in approximately 10% of patients with Down's syndrome (Fig. 3–5). The resultant atlantoaxial instability is detected by study of flexion and extension radiographs of the cervical spine taken in the lateral projection. With significant instability, the upper cervical spinal cord may be at risk of injury, and surgical fusion of C1 to C2 should be considered. Symptoms of C1–C2 instability include hyperreflexia, pain, and weakness.

Congenital occipitocervical fusion is a fibrous or osseous union between the atlas and the base of the occiput. This condition is usually associated with torticollis. It produces increased stress on the C1–C2 area, and instability may occur. Surgical extension of the fusion to C2 may be required.

Basilar impression occurs when the upper cervical spine appears to protrude into the foramen magnum. This may be a congenital anomaly, often associated with other cervical defects, or may occur as an acquired condition in patients with soft bones. Children with

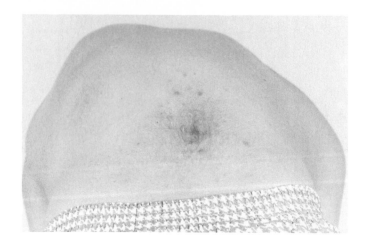

Figure 3–4. Left thoracic scoliosis with a left rib prominence on forward bending. Note the area of hypertrichosis in the thoracolumbar region. This patient also has a diastematomyelia in the low thoracic spine.

basilar impression appear to have a short neck, a low hairline, and often torticollis. It is frequently associated with other neurologic conditions, such as syringomyelia or the Arnold-Chiari malformation. Basilar impression is best detected by means of computerized tomography with reconstructed views. If neurologic deficit is present or impending or if spinal instability is detected on dynamic views, surgical treatment is warranted.

Several other variations of the odontoid process of the axis may occur, including os odontoideum, usually an ununited fracture, in which the odontoid appears to be a separate ossicle (Fig. 3–6); hypoplasia of the odontoid; and complete absence of the odontoid process. An abnormality in the region of the odontoid should be suspected in children who present with torticollis, with neurologic abnormality in the upper spinal cord, or with progressive neurologic deficit such as insidious weakness or irritability. In this or any other condition involving the atlantoaxial

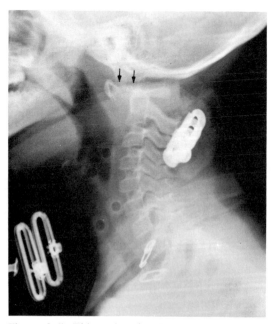

Figure 3–5. This patient has Down's syndrome and atlantoaxial instability. Note the anterior displacement of C1 relative to the odontoid process. A spinal fusion of C1 and C2 was required.

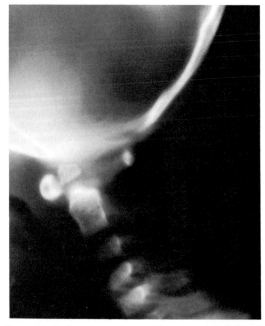

Figure 3–6. Os odontoideum. Note the lytic defect in the odontoid process.

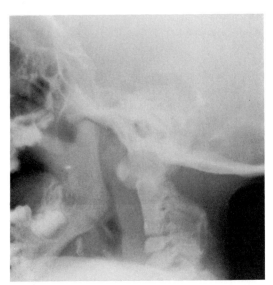

Figure 3–7. Klippel-Feil syndrome with fusion of the first four cervical vertebrae posteriorly and of C2 and C3 anteriorly.

junction, an indication for surgical fusion is proven C1–C2 instability.

The term "Klippel-Feil syndrome" is used to describe bony anomalies in the cervical spine. Part or all of the cervical spine may be involved with hemivertebrae, fused vertebrae, or other anomalies (Fig. 3–7). These children appear to have a short neck with a limited range of motion and a low hairline (Fig. 3–8). Torticollis, apparent neck webbing, plagiocephaly, and facial asymmetry may also be seen. Sprengel's deformity occurs in about one third of cases. Other associated findings include scoliosis or kyphosis (60% of cases), abnormalities of the urinary tract (30%), hearing loss (30%), and cardiac lesions (15%). The approach to a child with Klippel-Feil syndrome includes assessment of the cardiovascular system and the urinary tract, a neurologic evaluation and a careful search for other spinal abnormalities. Associated occipitocervical instability must be ruled out. Most frequently, patients with Klippel-Feil syndrome require no treatment other than periodic observation. In the rare cases in which adjacent cervical segments become unstable or painful, surgical fusion may be necessary.

Torticollis

Torticollis, or "wryneck," most often occurs as a benign cosmetic problem caused by tightness in one sternocleidomastoid muscle. The right side is more commonly involved than the left (Fig. 3–9). Such tightness is most

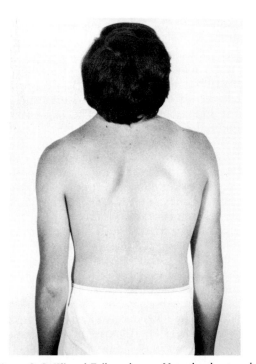

Figure 3–8. Klippel-Feil syndrome. Note the short neck, low hairline, and associated mild cervicothoracic scoliosis with shoulder asymmetry and slight left scapular prominence.

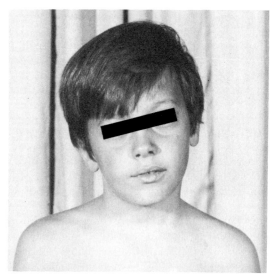

Figure 3–9. Congenital muscular torticollis with a tight right sternocleidomastoid muscle. Note that the patient's head deviates toward the involved side, with slight rotation of the chin away from the tight muscle.

often due to fibrosis in the muscle, which may occur because of a myopathy, denervation, venous occlusion, or pressure in utero or during delivery. It also may be caused by direct trauma, but this is very unlikely. Although common muscular torticollis responds readily to an exercise program during infancy or early childhood, there are other causes of torticollis for which exercises could be catastrophic. These include neoplasms and infections in the vertebral column, spinal cord, and soft tissues of the neck; traumatic fractures, subluxations, and dislocations of the upper cervical and atlantoocciptal region; and congenital cervical spine malformations. Clearly, all children with torticollis should undergo adequate radiographic examination of the neck, including an anteroposterior (AP) view and lateral flexion and extension views, to assess the stability and integrity of the cervical region. Other causes of torticollis include pterygii, congenital spinal cord lesions, ocular problems such as amblyopia, and gastroesophageal reflux. Common muscular torticollis may not be present in infancy but may arise de novo during childhood.

In congenital muscular torticollis with a tight sternocleidomastoid muscle, the head is tilted toward the involved side with the chin rotated toward the opposite shoulder. In early infancy, it is sometimes possible to palpate a mass in the involved muscle. This mass is felt to be representative of early organizing fibrosis and almost always contracts and disappears. If the condition does not resolve spontaneously with active stretching of the muscle by the infant, then plagiocephaly and facial asymmetry may develop. These are most likely caused by the position of the infant's head while sleeping. A supine sleeper develops flattening of the contralateral side of the skull, while a prone sleeper will show flattening of the ipsilateral side of the face.

An exercise program almost always corrects congenital muscular torticollis in children younger than one year old. The exercises are designed to place maximum distance between the ipsilateral sternoclavicular joint and mastoid process. This is accomplished by gently bending the neck laterally, away from the torticollis, and then slowly providing maximum rotation of the head and the face toward the side of the torticollis. This position should be held five seconds, released, and repeated five or 10 times. It is good to exercise at least four times a day or, better yet, at each diaper change. It may also be

helpful to position the infant in the crib in the prone position with the normal side toward the wall. This may cause some rotation toward the affected side and may help with the stretching program. If facial asymmetry is profound, if the child is older than two years of age, or if restriction of neck rotation exceeds 30 degrees compared with the normal side, then the exercises, while worth a try, will have a high failure rate. Surgery is then indicated, the most common procedure being a distal release of both the sternal and clavicular attachments of the muscle. Surgical results are not age dependent, and a good result may be expected in children up to and older than 10 years of age.

Finally, it is important to note that a 10% to 20% incidence of congenital hip dysplasia is associated with congenital muscular torticollis.

Congenital Scoliosis

Scoliosis in the neonate or infant may range from being undetectable to being quite severe. The structural basis for congenital scoliosis can be a failure of formation of vertebral structures (e.g., a wedged or triangular hemivertebra), a failure of segmentation (a unilateral bony or cartilaginous bar or fusion of adjacent asymmetric vertebrae), or combinations of formation and segmentation defects (Fig. 3–10). The significance of congenital scoliosis is that if it is undetected, severe deformities can develop and possibly affect visceral function, neurologic function, and cosmetic appearance. The existence of congenital scoliosis is suspected whenever one finds a recognizable deformity of the spine or trunk or a skin lesion present over the spinal column. The latter include cystic masses, hemangiomata, dimples, sinus tracts, hypertrichosis, and hyperpigmentation. Other musculoskeletal deformities, such as congenital hip dysplasia, lumbosacral agenesis, diastematomyelia, Klippel-Feil syndrome, Sprengel's deformity, and occipitocervical problems, are found more frequently in patients with congenital scoliosis.

Approximately 20% to 35% of children with congenital scoliosis will have anomalies of the urinary tract, making prompt evaluation of this system mandatory (Fig. 3–11). An increased incidence of congenital heart disease also coexists with congenital scoliosis.

The natural history of congenital scoliosis

depends upon the type of abnormality found. The worst prognosis is associated with a unilateral unsegmented bar. This in and of itself is an indication for prompt localized spinal fusion, since further growth will only increase the deformity, and there is no potential for longitudinal growth in such lesions. Multiple hemivertebrae on the same side of the spine also have a very poor prognosis and usually require surgical fusion. Isolated hemivertebrae and other mixed anomalies require careful observation to document progression before treatment is recommended. Overall, about 50% of all cases of congenital scoliosis will be progressive and require surgery.

When considering treatment for congenital scoliosis, two things must be kept in mind. First, it is a mistake to continue watching a progressive congenital scoliotic lesion. Further longitudinal growth will not occur; the patient will not become taller, only increasingly deformed. With progression of the curvature, the structurally involved segments should be promptly fused in situ to prevent

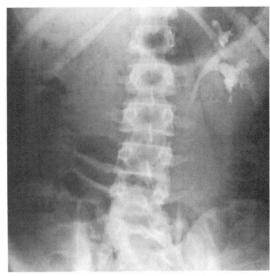

Figure 3–11. Unilateral agenesis of the right kidney in a patient with partial agenesis of the sacrum. Renal anomalies are extremely common in patients with congenital spinal malformations.

irretrievable deformity. Remember, a short but relatively straight spine is far better than a shorter, more deformed spine. The second consideration is the compensatory curve that usually develops above or below the structurally involved segment. Compensatory curves are sometimes amenable to brace control, since they are not fixed, rigid structures.

Congenital Kyphosis

Congenital kyphosis may occur as a severe angular deformity present at birth or may be an occult static or insidiously progressive angulation in the thoracic or thoracolumbar region (Fig. 3–12). One cause is the failure of formation of the anterior portion of the vertebral body at a single level or, less commonly, over short segments. This type is virtually always progressive and can lead to severe deformity and loss of neurologic function, even resulting in total paraplegia. A second cause is anterior fusion (failure of segmentation) of the vertebral bodies. In this situation, careful ongoing follow-up is mandatory, but uniform progression is not the rule.

With either type, brace treatment is completely ineffective and, therefore, contraindicated. Surgery is the only effective means of treatment and should be done as soon as

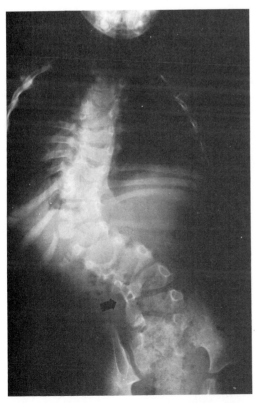

Figure 3–10. Congenital scoliosis with multiple anomalies of the spine. Note the unilateral bar in the left lower lumbar region *(arrow)*.

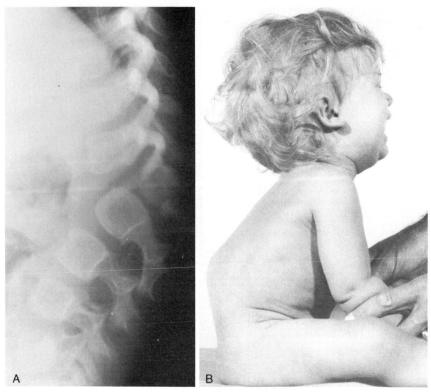

Figure 3–12. *A*, Congenital kyphosis secondary to failure of vertebral bodies to form at T12 and L1. *B*, The clinical appearance of the child. Thoracolumbar kyphosis is obvious.

indicated, even in early infancy. The two absolute indications are: (1) the presence of a posterior hemivertebra or failure of formation, and (2) progressive kyphosis due to failure of segmentation. The procedure of choice usually is a short posterior fusion to arrest posterior spinal growth and further progression of the deformity. When congenital kyphosis exceeds 50 degrees, posterior fusion alone is usually inadequate. In these cases, an anterior fusion, with or without excision of vertebral bodies, must be done before posterior fusion.

Caudal Spinal Agenesis

The syndrome of caudal agenesis or regression is manifested most often by sacral, lumbosacral, or, more rarely, isolated lumbar agenesis (Fig. 3–13). This condition is the failure of development of the caudal segments of the vertebral column and accompanying motor nerves. Sensation is intact, usually to at least the mid or lower sacral level. Although the cause is unknown, ap-

proximately 20% of the cases arise in offspring of diabetic mothers. Some teratogenic agents also have been implicated.

The clinical presentation of a child with this syndrome varies with the amount of agenesis. The severely involved child has a classic "buddha-like" appearance, with flexion and abduction contractures and webbing of the hips, knee flexion contractures with popliteal webbing, and severe foot deformities. The pelvis is narrow and foreshortened, the gluteal cleft is usually small or absent, and posterior dimpling over the hip joints is seen. The spectrum of clinical deformities ranges from severe involvement to partial sacral lesions, which may show a mild foot deformity as their only apparent defect.

Motor loss in spinal agenesis parallels the vertebral defect within one level, but sensation remains intact caudally for several segments. All but the most mildly afflicted patients will have a neurogenic bladder and bowel. Other congenital anomalies in the urinary tract and gastrointestinal system are common. The most common musculoskeletal

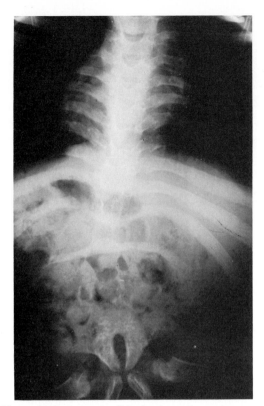

Figure 3–13. Agenesis of the lumbar spine and sacrum.

problems associated with caudal regression are scoliosis, foot deformity, major lower extremity joint contractures, and hip dysplasia or dislocation. Treatment is highly individualized and is best managed by specialized teams, such as those caring for patients with myelodysplasia. Surgical and orthotic treatment can be extremely beneficial to the child.

ACQUIRED SPINAL DISORDERS

Juvenile Hyperlordosis

Hyperlordosis or "swayback" is a common finding in the pediatric population, especially in girls before the onset of the adolescent growth spurt. The child appears to have an excessive amount of lumbar lordosis and an increased protuberance of the abdomen, an apparent potbelly. There may be a genetic predisposition, particularly in certain of the African population. The idiopathic type is thought to be caused by a period of relatively rapid skeletal growth unaccompanied by appropriate stretching of the posterior soft tissues, in particular the lumbar fascia and paraspinal muscles. This may have a tethering effect on the lumbar spine, producing hyperlordosis. Tightness of the hamstring muscles may be associated with this condition.

In the assessment of hyperlordosis, it is important to obtain a standing lateral radiograph of the entire spine in order to rule out other conditions, such as spondylolisthesis, as the underlying primary cause. Hyperlordosis also may be a compensatory mechanism below a structural thoracic hyperkyphosis or above femoral anteversion.

The appropriate radiographic measurement of lordosis is done with the Cobb method, measuring from the top of L1 to the top of S1. Normal values range from about 35 degrees to 65 degrees, depending upon the amount of sacral tilt.

The treatment for juvenile hyperlordosis is simple. It consists of an exercise program of trunk curls or partial sit-ups performed with the knees bent to relax the iliopsoas muscles and to exercise primarily the abdominal muscles while stretching the tight posterior structures. Twenty to 40 repetitions, performed once a day, are adequate. If the hamstrings are tight, appropriate stretching exercises for them are also advisable. The rare patient with idiopathic hyperlordosis who does not respond to an exercise program will respond readily to an antilordotic type of lumbar orthosis.

Idiopathic Scoliosis

Scoliosis is defined as a lateral curvature of the spine, usually associated with rotation of the vertebrae around their vertical axes. Such rotation is almost always with the posterior elements of the vertebrae rotated toward the concavity of the curve. The idiopathic type constitutes 80% to 85% of all cases. In this type, in contrast to congenital scoliosis, there are no primary structural anomalies in the vertebrae. The cause is probably multifactorial and includes subtle central nervous system dysfunction, genetic predisposition, and other factors.

The incidence of scoliosis in the adult population is approximately 4% if the most minor detectable curves are included. Approximately 0.3% (3 per 1000) of the population have curves that either have been or should have been treated.

Idiopathic scoliosis is divided into infantile, juvenile, and adolescent types. The infantile

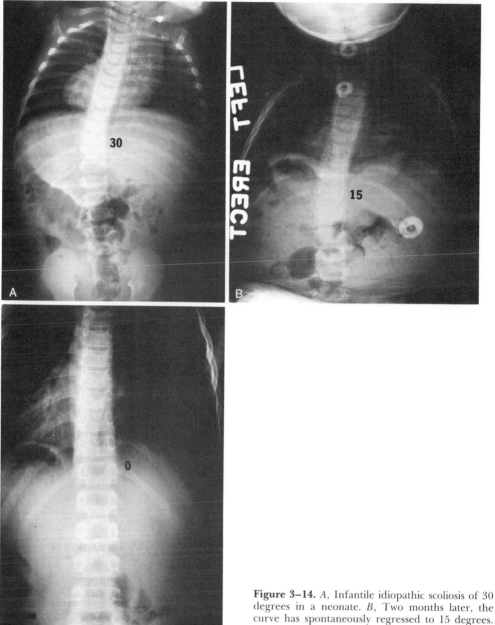

Figure 3–14. *A*, Infantile idiopathic scoliosis of 30 degrees in a neonate. *B*, Two months later, the curve has spontaneously regressed to 15 degrees. *C*, At eight years of age, the spine is essentially straight.

type arises before the age of three years but is not often detectable in infancy. This type is unusual in that spontaneous resolution of the curve occurs in 80% of the cases (Fig. 3–14). The work of Mehta has been helpful in forecasting which curves will be progressive. She has described a method for determining the rib–vertebral angle difference and the phase of overlap of the rib with the vertebral body. Using her criteria, progressive curves can be identified on the initial visit with better than 80% confidence. Infantile curves that are greater than 30 degrees at the time of presentation also have a propensity for progression.

Infantile idiopathic scoliosis is more common in boys and usually presents as a single curve, frequently over a long spinal segment. Curves greater than 30 degrees and curves showing definite progression should be treated with an appropriate orthosis. Spinal fusion is almost never a reasonable consideration in infantile idiopathic scoliosis because it arrests further growth of the spine. This is in contrast to progressing congenital scoliosis, for which spinal fusion is mandatory at any age.

Juvenile idiopathic scoliosis (onset at age three to nine years) and the adolescent type (onset at 10 years or older) behave differently from the infantile type. The remainder of this section deals with these types of scoliosis.

The diagnosis of idiopathic scoliosis is simple and is made by looking for five specific physical signs. These are easily detected by examining a child who is undressed from the waist up (Fig. 3–15). The child stands with back to the examiner, feet together, head up and looking straight ahead, and arms relaxed at the sides. The examiner looks for: (1) asymmetric shoulder levels, (2) prominence of one scapula, (3) unequal distances from the arms to the trunk or an unequal waistline, and (4) a palpable lateral curving of the spine. Next, the child bends forward at the waist with the arms dangling loosely forward (the Adams test). In this position the most reliable sign, an asymmetric prominence of one side of the chest or lumbar region, is detectable.

Because scoliosis in the juvenile or adolescent is painless and asymptomatic, and because children are rarely seen by their parents in an unclad state at that age, the school is the most appropriate place for comprehen-

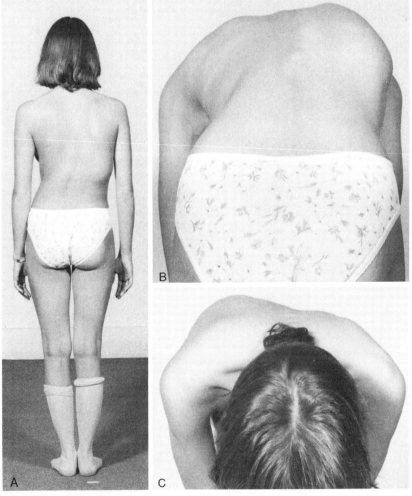

Figure 3–15. *A*, Adolescent idiopathic scoliosis viewed from the back. Note the right-sided thoracic prominence. When the patient bends forward, the rib prominence is even more apparent. This is secondary to rotation of the ribs and spine. *C*, When viewed from the front, the rib prominence is also quite evident.

sive screening programs. School screening is now mandatory in many areas of the United States and in several other countries.

Once scoliosis is suspected from a screening examination, all detected patients should have a standing posteroanterior radiographic examination of the entire spine, from the cervical region to the coccyx. This is necessary because spinal anomalies may be present and because balanced double structural idiopathic curves may be very difficult to detect. Remember that scoliosis is a physical sign, not a diagnosis (*idiopathic* scoliosis is a diagnosis), and for this reason thorough physical and neurologic examination, as well as radiologic confirmation, is essential initially for all patients who have scoliosis. It is also important to remember that idiopathic scoliosis does not cause pain. Children with painful scoliosis should be suspected of having a spinal tumor until proven otherwise.

Once the diagnosis of idiopathic scoliosis is confirmed, then ongoing follow-up is necessary. It is most appropriate for pediatricians, family physicians, and nurse practitioners to continue following those patients who do not need active treatment. This would include most of those children with curves of less than 25 degrees. Idiopathic curves that are progressing or are greater than 25 degrees, or both, should be referred to an orthopedic surgeon who is knowledgeable in the treatment of scoliosis.

At present, there are only three rational and proven effective means of treating progressive idiopathic scoliosis: a surgical procedure, an orthosis, or a neuromuscular stimulator (Fig. 3–16). The specifics of the various types of orthoses and stimulators are beyond the scope of this text. Suffice it to say, however, that other modalities such as spinal manipulation, traction, exercise programs, megavitamin therapy, diets, and so forth have never been shown to be effective in altering the natural course of scoliosis and may, in fact, be harmful by allowing relentless curve progression to occur under the false blanket of "doing something."

The medical significance of scoliosis depends upon the location and magnitude of the curve. Thoracic curves that exceed 60 degrees can produce significant restrictive and obstructive pulmonary disease and subsequent cor pulmonale. When these curves approach 90 degrees, significantly decreased longevity is expected. Curves in the thoraco-

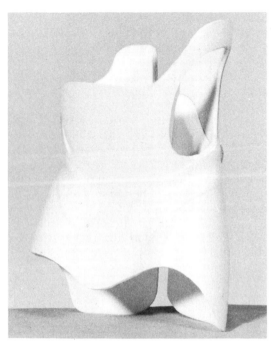

Figure 3–16. This type of modular low-profile spinal orthosis is currently in use in many centers for the treatment of idiopathic scoliosis.

lumbar and lumbar regions do not affect pulmonary function very much but do have the propensity for causing increased low back pain in adult life. It is best to attempt to restrict a curve to less than 30 to 40 degrees if at all possible. Additionally, the larger the curve, irrespective of its location, the greater is the likelihood of cosmetic deformity.

Although all curves are individual problems, and totally accurate prediction of future curve behavior is impossible, certain guidelines for progression are known. A safe generalization is that the younger the child and the greater the magnitude of the curve, the greater is the risk of progression. It is known that some curves, particularly those greater than 40 to 50 degrees, may continue progressing at variable rates throughout life. The axiom that *all* curves stop progressing at skeletal maturity is a myth, although it is unusual for a curve of less than 30 degrees to continue increasing beyond the end of growth. Of note is the fact that although very rare, some curves arise de novo in adults.

Orthotic treatment or neuromuscular stimulation is appropriate for progressing curves that exceed 25 to 30 degrees in immature individuals (Fig. 3–17). The upper range of successful nonoperative treatment is usually

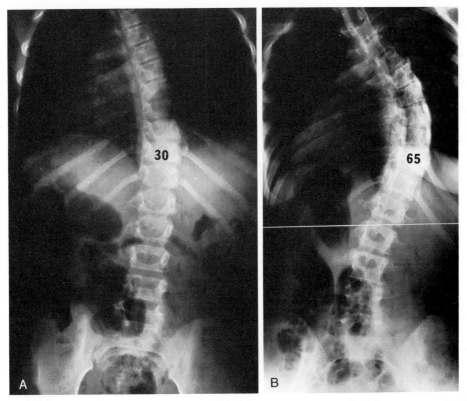

Figure 3–17. *A,* Mild idiopathic scoliosis in a 10-year-old girl. A brace was prescribed but not worn. *B,* The curve progressed to a more severe magnitude, and spinal fusion was required.

40 to 45 degrees. Above this magnitude in growing children progression is often the rule, either during or after treatment, and surgery should be considered (Figs. 3–18 and 3–19).

Adolescent Kyphosis

Abnormal kyphosis is defined as excessive roundback of the thoracic spine. It is measured by the method of Cobb from the most tilted upper thoracic vertebra, usually T1, to the inferior end-plate of the most tilted lower vertebra, usually T12. Measurement is done from a standing lateral radiograph. It is important to measure the maximally tilted vertebrae, which may not always be T1 and T12. The normal angle ranges from 20 to 45 degrees.

Hyperkyphosis has a propensity to become rigid and may be progressive beyond adolescence and into adulthood. A rigid hyperkyphosis may cause back pain, easy fatigability, pulmonary compromise, and cosmetic de-

formity. It is extremely rare for it to reach such a degree as to cause neurologic deficit from anterior pressure on the spinal cord. The incidence of hyperkyphosis in school-aged children is approximately 4% in the United States. On clinical examination, it is best detected by viewing a forward-bending child from the side. In the abnormal case, posteriorly directed angulation is seen instead of a smooth gentle arc (Fig. 3–20).

There are two types of hyperkyphosis seen in the pediatric population. One is postural roundback, which has excessive curvature but no vertebral changes. The distribution of this type is about equal between the sexes. The second type, more common in boys, is Scheuermann's disease, which is defined as hyperkyphosis with structural vertebral changes, including greater than five degrees of wedging in at least two or three consecutive vertebrae. End-plate irregularities of the vertebral bodies and intervertebral disc space narrowing are often seen (Fig. 3–21). In contrast to those with postural roundback, which is usually painless, approximately 40%

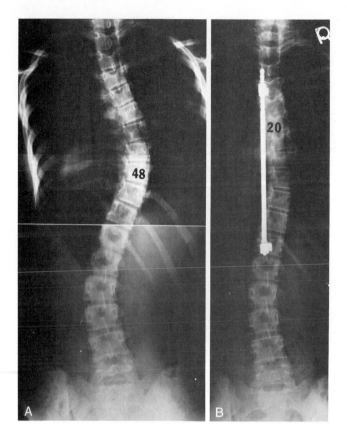

Figure 3–18. *A*, Forty-eight-degree right thoracic scoliosis in a 12-year-old girl. *B*, The patient was treated with Harrington instrumentation and posterior spinal fusion. The curve has been reduced to 20 degrees.

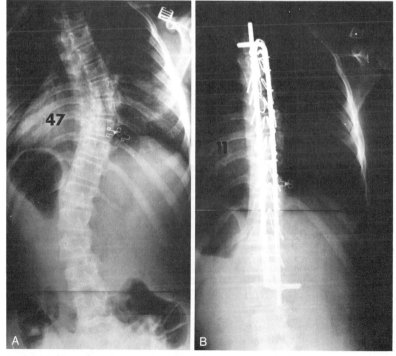

Figure 3–19. *A*, Forty-seven-degree right thoracic scoliosis in a 12-year-old girl. *B*, This patient underwent posterior spinal fusion utilizing L-rod segmental instrumentation. Her curve was corrected to 11 degrees.

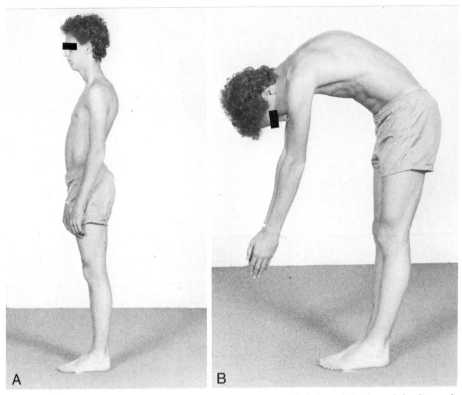

A   B

Figure 3–20. *A,* Adolescent kyphosis. Note the lumbar lordosis, the rounded thoracic back, and the forward projection of the head and neck. *B,* When the patient bends forward, the angular deformity in the midthoracic spine is apparent.

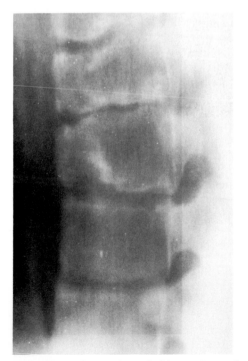

Figure 3–21. End-plate irregularities and vertebral wedging consistent with Scheuermann's disease.

to 50% of patients with Scheuermann's disease complain of localized back pain. Scheuermann's disease usually occurs in the midthoracic or thoracolumbar regions. The probable cause is relative osteopenia or structural insufficiency of the vertebral end-plates, probably related to rapid overall skeletal growth, which allows micro- or macro-compression of the vertebral bodies.

The treatment for mild hyperkyphosis consists of either observation or thoracic hyperextension and lumbar antilordotic exercises. For larger curves not greater than 75 to 80 degrees, an orthosis plus an exercise program is appropriate (Fig. 3–22). The type of orthosis may be either a low profile type or a full Milwaukee brace. Occasionally, dramatic improvement from orthotic treatment can be seen in kyphosis as great as 80 degrees, provided that the patient is skeletally immature. Since the growth plates of the thoracic vertebrae are among the last in the spine to close (at about 17 years of age in females and 19 years in males), orthotic treatment may be successful even though the remainder of the patient's skeleton is mature.

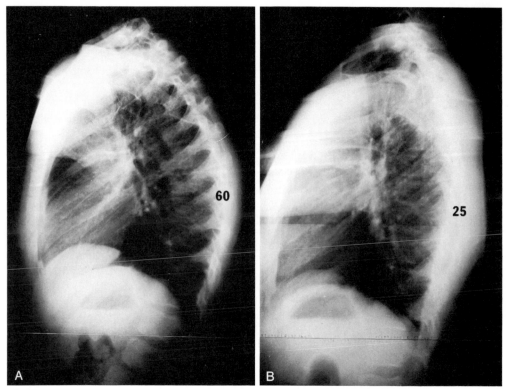

Figure 3–22. *A,* Pretreatment lateral radiograph of postural round back. The patient's kyphotic curve measured 60 degrees. *B,* Posttreatment radiograph. The kyphosis is now 25 degrees. The patient was treated with a Milwaukee brace.

Surgery may be appropriate for some patients who have more than 70 degrees of kyphosis and who are fully skeletally mature (Fig. 3–23). Another indication for surgical correction is a short, sharply angled kyphosis, regardless of magnitude. This type is likely to progress or to become painful or both. Surgical correction is a safe, reasonable treatment alternative and is far preferable to allowing an individual to go through life with severe deformity and the risk of pain and continued progression.

Spondylolisthesis

Spondylolisthesis is the slipping forward of one vertebra upon another. It has been subclassified into five types: dysplastic, isthmic, degenerative, traumatic, and pathologic. Only the first two types are commonly found in children and adolescents. Both result from a lesion at the pars interarticularis of the posterior vertebral arch. In the dysplastic type, this portion of the bone becomes elongated, whereas in the isthmic type, a fatigue fracture occurs with subsequent failure to heal (Figs. 3–24 and 3–25). Because of this, the vertebral articulation is weakened, and the cephalad vertebral body is free to slide forward (spondylolisthesis) on the more caudal one. The dysplastic type may also result from abnormal development of the cephalad position of the body of the first sacral vertebra.

Spondylolisthesis is most common at the lumbosacral junction and occurs with progressively decreasing frequency at L4, L3, L2, and L1. It is rarely seen in children younger than the age of five years. The isthmic fatigue fracture, known as spondylolysis, occurs in about 5% of the American population. Approximately half of these will progress to spondylolisthesis.

The pars fatigue fracture results from forced flexion or forced rotation of the lumbar spine and, therefore, is common in young gymnasts and in football players. In the isthmic type, there is a family history in about 15%, and spina bifida occulta at the involved vertebral level is seen in one third of the cases. The dysplastic type is less common but is associated with a positive family history in

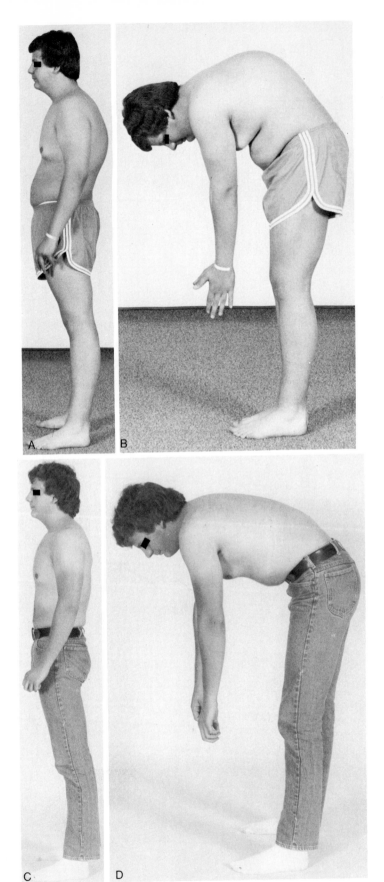

Figure 3–23. Pre- (A, B) and postoperative (C, D) views of an adolescent male with severe kyphosis secondary to Scheuermann's disease. He required both anterior and posterior spinal fusion. He now has a markedly improved appearance and no further progression of the kyphosis.

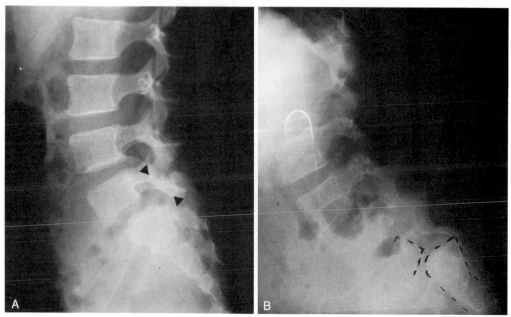

Figure 3–24. *A,* Spondylolisthesis of L5 on S1 secondary to dysplastic elongation of the pars interarticularis. *B,* Observation documented further forward slipping and rotation of L5 on S1. This patient required spinal fusion.

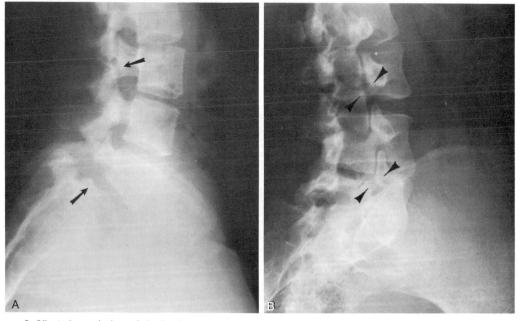

Figure 3–25. *A,* Lateral view of the lumbar spine showing spondylolysis at L5, with a mild slip of L5 on S1 *(lower arrow).* The upper arrow shows a subtle defect at L3. *B,* An oblique projection of the same patient. Both areas of spondylolysis are clearly seen.

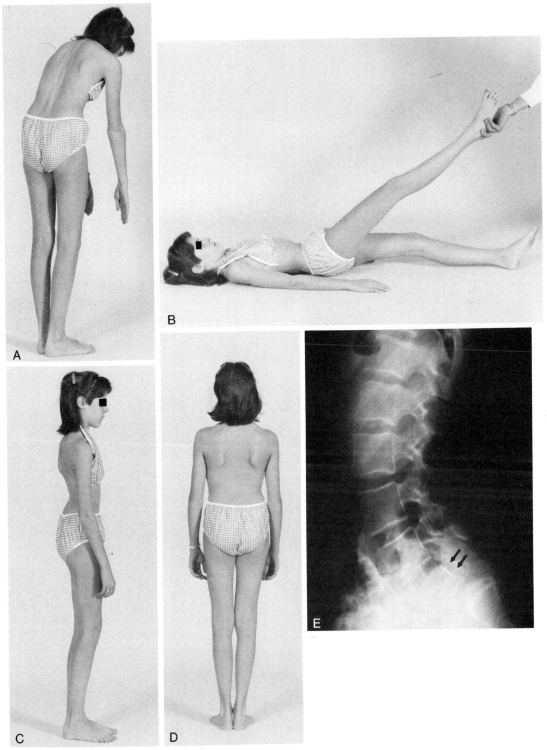

Figure 3–26. *A,* This patient demonstrates the physical findings of severe spondylolisthesis. There is marked limitation of forward flexion of the spine, with paraspinal spasm in the lumbar muscles and tightness of the hamstrings. *B,* This allows the straight-leg to raise to only 40 degrees. *C,* She also demonstrates accentuated lumbar lordosis and a short trunk. *D,* Mild scoliosis is present as well with flattening of the left waistline. *E,* Radiograph of this patient.

33%. Spina bifida occulta is associated about 95% of the time. Conservative therapy will fail more often with the dysplastic than with the isthmic type, and surgical treatment will be required.

Spondylolisthesis occurs only in humans. It has never been seen in nonambulatory patients and is the most common cause of back pain in adolescents. The signs and symptoms may include low back, buttock, and thigh pain, which rarely goes below the knee; tight hamstrings; postural deformity with hyperlordosis and, in the severe grades, a palpable "step-off" at the lumbosacral junction; mild weakness and hypesthesia in the lower extremities; and abnormalities of gait (Fig. 3–26). The diagnosis is confirmed by means of plain radiographs, including a standing posteroanterior (PA) and lateral view and oblique views to define the condition of the pars interarticularis. The PA view should include the entire spine, since scoliosis is associated with this condition about 40% of the time.

Once spondylolisthesis has been detected, even patients who are asymptomatic should be followed. There is a small but definite risk of increased slipping, particularly before the age of 15. The risk of a progressive slip is independent of the initial magnitude of the slip, and it is more likely in the immature spine with dysplastic changes and in the child whose sacrum is more vertically oriented than usual. Although progressive slipping can lead to neurologic deficit, from which recovery may not occur (even with prompt treatment), this is exceedingly rare. The question of whether the asymptomatic patient with spondylolysis or mild spondylolisthesis as an incidental finding should be allowed to participate in contact sports often arises. Most orthopedic surgeons do not categorically forbid such participation.

Nonoperative treatment of symptomatic spondylolisthesis may include limiting activity, bed rest, nonnarcotic analgesics, and perhaps a trial of immobilization in a cast or orthosis. Acute spondylolysis, a pars interarticularis fracture seen following trauma, demands immobilization and will usually heal within a period of three months.

Unfortunately, conservative treatment does not often succeed in patients with the chronic types of painful spondylolisthesis. The indications for surgery are refractory pain, progressive slipping, severe deformity (greater than a 50% slip relative to the adja-cent vertebra), or a significant gait disturbance. Surgical treatment most often consists of a bilateral transverse process spinal fusion, from L4 or L5 to the sacrum. The results of surgical treatment are quite good, with more than 95% of patients being asymptomatic and able to return to an active life, including vigorous athletic activities, once the fusion has consolidated and matured.

BACK PAIN IN CHILDREN AND ADOLESCENTS

Although the incidence of back pain in children and adolescents is far less than in the adult population, such pain is more likely to be based on a major pathologic lesion than on chronic muscular or ligamentous strain or early degenerative changes. Although spondylolisthesis is the most common cause of low back pain in adolescents, nevertheless it is essential to consider that any child complaining of back pain may have a tumor (neoplasm), herniated disc, or infection of the spine or spinal cord until proven otherwise (Fig. 3–27). Such mass lesions have the potential to produce permanent neurologic deficit and spinal destruction unless promptly diagnosed and treated. Only after all other causes have been ruled out can the diagnosis of a muscular or ligamentous strain, or of a functional or hysterical cause of back pain, be justified.

Neoplasms

Neoplasms of the spine or neural axis usually present with pain that is often constant in nature, involuntary muscle spasm, rigidity of the spine on attempted active motion, and neurologic deficit. Neurologic deficit may include weakness, sensory deficit, foot deformity, or interference with bowel or bladder control. Once the diagnosis of a neoplasm has been established, prompt surgical treatment is indicated for almost all lesions. An exception would be eosinophilic granuloma, which often runs a self-limited course or may respond to low-dose radiation therapy. It is confirmed by means of a needle biopsy.

Infections

Back pain caused by infection of the spinal column is usually due to discitis (infection in

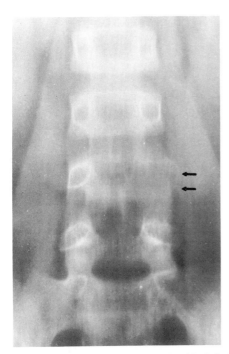

Figure 3–27. This patient presented with left-sided lumbar back pain. Note the destruction of the vertebral pedicle at L4. This proved to be an osteoblastoma. Children with back pain should be suspected of having a tumor of the spine or spinal cord until proven otherwise.

the intervertebral disc space) in children and adolescents (Fig. 3–28). Vertebral osteomyelitis is a disease that occurs mostly in adults. The reason for this is the ontogeny of the blood supply to the spinal column. Discitis results from hematogenous seeding from a bacteremia, with the primary source of infection being in the respiratory or urinary tract in most cases. Sixty per cent of all disc space infections occur in children younger than the age of six years. They occur most commonly in the lumbar region and are usually caused by *Staphylococcus aureus*. The clinical presentation consists of back pain, commonly with pain radiating to the hip or leg. Occasional cases present as isolated abdominal pain, or simply as a limp or refusal or inability to walk. Tenderness to percussion over the involved area of the spine and involuntary myospasm are common. Fever may be present or absent. The white blood count is often mildly to moderately increased but may be normal, and the erythrocyte sedimentation rate is always increased. Blood cultures or aspiration from the disc space, or both, will yield the causative organism in the majority

of cases. Plain radiographic views in discitis usually show positive findings after three weeks of symptoms. Initially, they show narrowing of the disc space, followed later by irregularity or erosions of the end-plate and often a soft tissue mass in the adjoining area. Radionuclide bone and soft tissue scans have positive findings much earlier.

Treatment of discitis consists of bed rest with or without a body cast, depending on the amount of back pain. Antibiotics are usually not necessary. The vast majority of cases respond to rest alone with subsiding of the symptoms and healing of the lesion. If progress toward healing, with resolution of the increased white cell count and sedimentation rate and disappearance of pain and spasm, has not occurred within two to three weeks, then aspiration of the disc space and institution of antibiotic treatment are indicated. Treatment should be continued until the sedimentation rate is normal. In painful cases, an extension body cast is helpful.

Although vertebral osteomyelitis is an adult disease, it can occur in children, particularly in debilitated adolescents or those who are frequent drug abusers. This infection presents with signs and symptoms similar to those of discitis, but radiographs show erosion and collapse of the vertebral body (Fig. 3–29). The treatment is different. When vertebral osteomyelitis is suspected, a needle biopsy to develop a culture of the lesion should be obtained and antibiotic treatment started promptly. Patients who do not respond to bed rest, immobilization in a cast, and antibiotics may be candidates for open surgical excisional biopsy and anterior spinal fusion.

Herniated Disc

An uncommon but well-recognized cause of back pain in children is a herniated disc. This presents a clinical picture similar to that seen in the adult, with back pain and radiculopathy. The pain radiates through the distribution of the sciatic nerve or a specific nerve root. A history of significant trauma is not always found with this lesion. A decreased range of spinal motion and involuntary muscle spasm are common. With significant nerve root compression, changes such as muscle weakness, atrophy, sensory loss, and reflex diminution are seen. Plain radiographs usually show normal findings, the

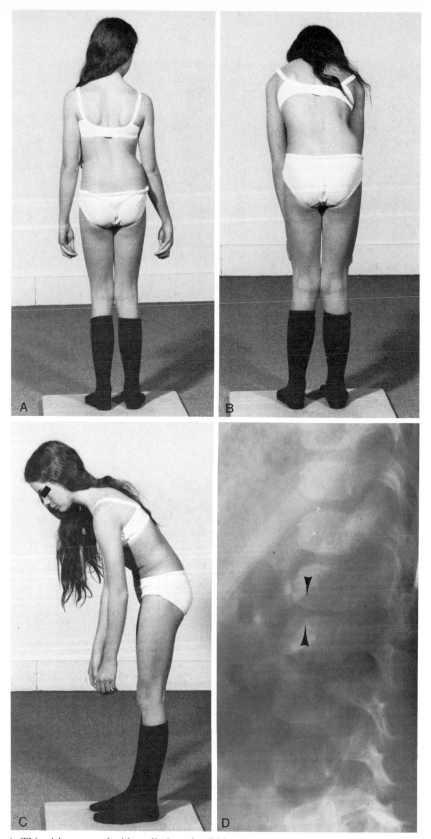

Figure 3–28. *A,* This girl presented with scoliosis and mild low back pain. *B* and *C,* Note the marked restriction of forward bending. This was caused by lumbar muscle spasm. It should arouse suspicion of a mass lesion in the spine. *D,* On radiographic examination, a disc space infection was found between L1 and L2.

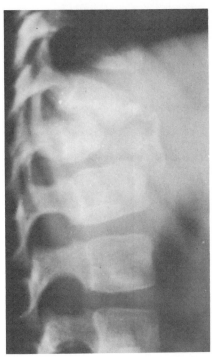

Figure 3–29. Osteomyelitis at T11 and T12. Note the destruction of the disc space and vertebral bodies with beginning of anterior ossification. This patient went on to spontaneous fusion and is now asymptomatic.

diagnosis being established by means of computerized tomography or myelography, or both (Fig. 3–30). The treatment of herniated disc disease in the pediatric population con-

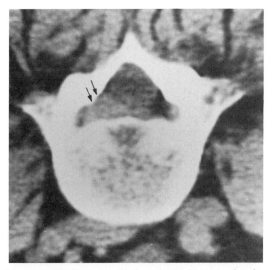

Figure 3–30. Computerized tomographic scan showing a large bulging disc on the left. Note the displacement of the dural sac.

sists initially of bed rest and administration of nonnarcotic analgesics for three to six weeks. An exception to this is the patient with a progressing neurologic deficit, who should have prompt surgical decompression with removal of the offending disc material. Another indication for surgical treatment is intractability with failure to respond to an adequate trial of conservative therapy. Surgical treatment classically involves a small laminectomy and excision of the disc material. Enzymatic injection treatment of the herniated disc with chymopapain or collagenase, while used in adults, is not recommended for children at present.

Back Strain

People who are prone to obesity or inactivity, or both—whether children or adults—frequently experience chronic muscular or ligamentous strain and low back pain. In children this is a "diagnosis of exclusion," other forms of more serious disease having been ruled out. The pain is nagging but tolerable, usually is intermittent, and rarely radiates. It responds best to muscle stretching and strengthening exercises, weight reduction, and alteration of activities until the patient is symptom-free.

Functional Back Pain

A final cause of back pain in children is hysteria or a conversion reaction. These patients present with bizarre somatic pain patterns. The results of a physical examination, including a meticulous neurologic evaluation, are completely normal. All laboratory and radiographic study results are normal. The child with functional back pain almost always shows disproportionate disability and an unusual affect, in addition to the bizarre somatic pattern. Treatment consists of attention to the psychosocial problems, not only of the patient, but also of the family.

References

Spina Bifida Occulta

Anderson FM: Occult spinal dysraphism: A series of 73 cases. Pediatrics 55:826, 1975.
Sutow WW and Pryde AW: Incidence of spina bifida occulta in relation to age. Am J Dis Child 91:211, 1956.

Myelomeningocele

American Academy of Orthopaedic Surgeons: Symposium on Myelomeningocele. St. Louis, CV Mosby Co, 1972.

Barden GA et al.: Myelodysplastics—fate of those followed for twenty years or more. J Bone Joint Surg 57A:643, 1975.

Hoffer MM et al.: Functional ambulation in patients with myelomeningocele. J Bone Joint Surg 55A:137, 1973.

Kilfoyle RM: Myelodysplasia. Pediatr Clin North Am 14:419, 1967.

Laurence KM: The natural history of spina bifida cystica: Detailed analysis of 407 cases. Arch Dis Child 39:41, 1964.

Lorber J: Results of treatment of myelomeningocele, an analysis of 524 unselected cases with special reference to possible selection for treatment. Dev Med Child Neurol, 13:279, 1971.

Diastematomyelia

Hilal SK and Martond-Pollack E: Diastematomyelia in children. Radiographic study of 34 cases. Radiology 112:609, 1974.

Winter RB et al.: Diastematomyelia and congenital spine deformities. J Bone Joint Surg 56A:27, 1974.

Cervical Spine Instability

Cattell H: Normal variations in cervical spine in children. J Bone Joint Surg 47A:1309, 1965.

Cattell H and Filtzer DL: Pseudosubluxation and other normal variations in the cervical spine in children. J Bone Joint Surg 47A:1295, 1965.

Dawson EG and Smith L: Atlantoaxial subluxation in children due to vertebral anomalies. J Bone Joint Surg 61A:582, 1979.

Fielding JW et al.: Os odontoideum. J Bone Joint Surg 62A:376, 1980.

Fielding JW and Hawkins RJ: Atlantoaxial rotatory fixation (fixed rotatory subluxation of the atlantoaxial joint). J Bone Joint Surg 59A:37, 1977.

Holmes JC and Hall JE: Fusion for instability and potential instability of the cervical spine in children and adolescents. Orthop Clin North Am 9:923, 1978.

Koop SE et al.: The surgical treatment of instability of the upper part of the cervical spine in children and adolescents. J Bone Joint Surg 66A:403, 1984.

Nicholson JT and Sherk HH: Anomalies of the occipitocervical articulation. J Bone Joint Surg 50A:295, 1968.

Spierings EL and Braakman R: The management of os odontoideum: Analysis of 37 cases. J Bone Joint Surg 64B:422, 1982.

Teodori JB and Painter MG: Basilar impression in children. Pediatrics 74:1097, 1984.

Yasuoka S et al.: The incidence of spinal deformity and instability after multiple level laminectomy: Its difference in children and adults. Orthop Trans 6:11, 1982.

Klippel-Feil Syndrome

Baird TA et al.: Klippel-Feil syndrome. Am J Dis Child 113:546, 1967.

Fietti VG Jr and Fielding JW: The Klippel-Feil syndrome: Early roentgenographic appearance and progression of the deformity. J Bone Joint Surg 58A:891, 1976.

Hensinger RN et al.: The Klippel-Feil syndrome—a constellation of related anomalies. J Bone Joint Surg 56A:1246, 1974.

Torticollis

Canale ST et al.: Congenital muscular torticollis. A long-term follow-up. J Bone Joint Surg 64A:810, 1982.

Coventry MB and Harris LE: Congenital muscular torticollis in infancy: Some observations regarding treatment. J Bone Joint Surg 41A:815, 1959.

Hummer C Jr and MacEwen GD: The co-existence of torticollis and congenital dysplasia of the hip. J Bone Joint Surg 54A:1255, 1972.

Ling CM: The influence of age on the results of open sternomastoid tenotomy in muscular torticollis. Clin Orthop 116:142, 1976.

Ling CM and Low YS: Sternomastoid tumor and muscular torticollis. Clin Orthop 86:144, 1972.

Morrison DL and MacEwen GD: Congenital muscular torticollis: Observations regarding clinical findings, associated conditions, and results of treatment. J Pediatr Orthop 2:500, 1982.

Sarant JB and Morrissy RT: Idiopathic torticollis: Sternocleidomastoid myopathy and accessory neuropathy. Muscle Nerve 4:374, 1981.

Congenital Scoliosis

Gillespie R et al.: Intraspinal anomalies in congenital scoliosis. Clin Orthop 93:103, 1973.

MacEwen GD et al.: Evaluation of kidney anomalies in congenital scoliosis. J Bone Joint Surg 54A:1451, 1972.

McMaster MJ and Ohtsuka K: The natural history of congenital scoliosis: A study of 251 patients. J Bone Joint Surg 64A:1128, 1982.

Winter RB: Congenital Deformities of the Spine. New York, Thieme-Stratton Inc, 1983.

Winter RB: Convex anterior and posterior hemi-arthrodesis and hemi-epiphyseodesis in young children with progressive congenital scoliosis. J Pediatr Orthop 1:361, 1981.

Winter RB and Moe JH: The results of spinal arthrodesis for congenital spine deformity in patients younger than 5 years old. J Bone Joint Surg 64A:419, 1982.

Congenital Kyphosis

Montgomery S and Hall J: Congenital kyphosis: Surgical treatment at Boston Children's Hospital. Orthop Trans 5:25, 1981.

Winter RB: Congenital kyphosis. Clin Orthop 128:26, 1977.

Winter RB et al.: Congenital kyphosis. Its natural history and treatment as observed in the study of 130 patients. J Bone Joint Surg 55A:223, 1973.

Sacral Agenesis

Andrish J et al.: Sacral agenesis: A clinical evaluation of its management, heredity, and associated anomalies. Clin Orthop 139:52, 1979.

Banta JV and Nichols O: Sacral agenesis. J Bone Joint Surg 51A:693, 1969.

Frantz CH and Aitken GT: Complete absence of the lumbar spine and sacrum. J Bone Joint Surg 49A:1531, 1967.

Phillips WA et al.: Orthopaedic management of lumbosacral agenesis. J Bone Joint Surg 64A:1282, 1982.

Renshaw TS: Sacral agenesis: A classification and review of 23 cases. J Bone Joint Surg 60A:373, 1978.

Idiopathic Scoliosis

Bjure J and Nachemson A: Non-treated scoliosis. Clin Orthop 93:44, 1973.

Blount WP and Mellencamp DD: The effect of pregnancy on idiopathic scoliosis. J Bone Joint Surg 62A:1083, 1980.

Carr WA et al.: Treatment of idiopathic scoliosis in the Milwaukee brace, long-term results. J Bone Joint Surg 62A;599, 1980.

Chong KC et al.: Influence of spinal curvature on exercise capacity. J Pediatr Orthop 1:251, 1981.

Dickson JH and Harrington PR: The evolution of the Harrington instrumentation technique in scoliosis. J Bone Joint Surg 55A:993, 1973.

Jacobs RR (ed): Pathogenesis of Idiopathic Scoliosis. Chicago, Scoliosis Research Society, 1984.

Lloyd-Roberts GC and Pilcher MF: Structural idiopathic scoliosis in infancy—a study of the natural history of 100 patients. J Bone Joint Surg 47B:520, 1965.

Lonstein JE et al.: Voluntary school screening for scoliosis in Minnesota. J Bone Joint Surg 64A:481, 1982.

Mehta MH: Infantile idiopathic scoliosis. J Bone Joint Surg 54B:230, 1972.

Mehta MH: The rib-vertebra angle in the early diagnosis between resolving and progressive infantile scoliosis. J Bone Joint Surg 54B:230, 1973.

Moe JH et al.: Scoliosis and Other Deformities. Philadelphia, WB Saunders Co, 1978.

Moe JH and Kettleson DN: Idiopathic scoliosis. Analysis of curve patterns and the preliminary results of Milwaukee brace treatment in 169 patients. J Bone Joint Surg 52A:1509, 1970.

Moskowitz A et al.: Long-term follow-up of scoliosis fusion. J Bone Joint Surg 62A:364, 1980.

Nachemson A: Adult scoliosis and back pain. Spine 4:513, 1979.

Nilsonne U and Lundgren K: Long-term prognosis in idiopathic scoliosis. Acta Orthop Scand 39:456, 1968.

Rogala EJ et al.: Scoliosis: Incidence and natural history, a prospective epidemiological study. J Bone Joint Surg 60A:173, 1978.

Stone B et al.: The effect of an exercise program on change in curve in adolescents with minimal idiopathic scoliosis. Phys Ther 59:759, 1979.

Torell G et al.: The changing pattern of scoliosis treatment due to effective screening. J Bone Joint Surg 63A:337, 1981.

Weinstein S et al.: Idiopathic scoliosis: Long-term follow-up and prognosis in untreated patients. J Bone Joint Surg 63A:702, 1981.

Yamada K et al.: Etiology of idiopathic scoliosis. Clin Orthop 184:50, 1984.

Adolescent Kyphosis

Bradford DS: Juvenile kyphosis. Clin Orthop 128:45, 1977.

Bradford DS et al.: Scheuermann's kyphosis and roundback deformity—results of Milwaukee brace treatment. J Bone Joint Surg 56A:740, 1974.

Bradford DS et al.: Scheuermann's kyphosis, a form of osteoporosis? Clin Orthop 118:10, 1976.

Bradford DS et al.: The surgical management of patients with Scheuermann's disease: A review of 24 cases managed by combined anterior and posterior spine fusion. J Bone Joint Surg 62A:705, 1980.

Montgomery SP and Erwin WE: Scheuermann's kyphosis—long-term results of Milwaukee brace treatment. Spine 6:5, 1981.

Spondylolisthesis

Boxall D et al.: Management of severe spondylolisthesis in children and adolescents. J Bone Joint Surg 61A:479, 1979.

Fredrickson BE et al.: The natural history of spondylolysis and spondylolisthesis. J Bone Joint Surg 66A:699, 1984.

Hensinger RN: Spondylolysis and spondylolisthesis in children. American Academy of Orthopaedic Surgeons Instructional Course Lectures 32:132, 1983.

Newman PH: The etiology of spondylolisthesis. J Bone Joint Surg 45B:39, 1963.

Sherman FC et al.: Spine fusion for spondylolysis and spondylolisthesis in children. Spine 4:59, 1979.

Turner RH and Bianco AJ Jr: Spondylolysis and spondylolisthesis in children and teenagers. J Bone Joint Surg 53A:1298, 1971.

Wiltse LL et al.: Classification of spondylolysis and spondylolisthesis. Clin Orthop 117:23, 1976.

Back Pain

Micheli LJ: Low back pain in the adolescent: Differential diagnosis. Am J Sports Med 7:362, 1979.

Tachdjian MO and Matson DD: Orthopaedic aspects of intraspinal tumors in infants and children. J Bone Joint Surg 47A:223, 1965.

Spinal Infections

Boston HC Jr et al.: Disk space infections in children. Orthop Clin North Am 6:953, 1975.

Eismont FJ et al.: Vertebral osteomyelitis in infants. J Bone Joint Surg 64B:32, 1982.

Peterson HA: Fungal osteomyelitis in children. American Academy of Orthopaedic Surgeons Instructional Course Lectures 32:46, 1983.

Reports of the Medical Research Council Working Party on Tuberculosis of the Spine. J Bone Joint Surg 58B:399, 1976; J Bone Joint Surg 60B:163, 1978; J Bone Joint Surg 64B:393, 1982.

Wenger DR et al.: The spectrum of intervertebral disk space infection in children. J Bone Joint Surg 60A:100, 1978.

Intervertebral Disc Lesions

Bulos S: Herniated intervertebral lumbar disk in the teenager. J Bone Joint Surg 55D:273, 1973.

Clarke NMP and Cleak DK: Intervertebral lumbar disc prolapse in children and adolescents. J Pediatr Orthop 3:202, 1983.

Nelson CL et al.: Disk protrusions in the young. Clin Orthop 88:142, 1972.

Sonnabend DH et al.: Intervertebral disk calcification syndromes in children. J Bone Joint Surg 64B:25, 1982.

4

The Hip

The hip is a major weight-bearing joint and must function well for satisfactory standing, walking, and running to occur. The normally functioning hip is free of pain and stable but mobile, although a painless, surgically fused hip can provide very good walking ability. The implications of unrecognized hip disease and subsequent permanent hip damage include pain, a limp, loss of motion, instability, shortening of the lower extremity, and an increased energy requirement during walking.

The hip lies deep within an envelope of skin, fat, connective tissue, and muscle and, therefore, does not display its condition as readily as do the arm and hand, or the leg and foot. Consequently, one must become an expert at the careful examination of the hip and make it a routine part of all pediatric physical evaluations. This chapter addresses the more common pediatric hip problems.

CONGENITAL DYSPLASIA OF THE HIP

Congenital dysplasia of the hip (CDH) describes a spectrum of kinds of abnormal development of the hip joint. It can range from barely detectable deviation from stable congruity of the femoral head in the depth of the acetabulum to unreducible dislocation with advanced adaptive changes. Thus, the diagnostic signs of CDH are variable, not only from patient to patient, but also during succeeding stages of development in the same patient. Abnormal findings in the neonatal period may disappear after the first few weeks of life, while other signs, which may be readily apparent when the child begins walking, may have been undetectable during infancy. When very mild but progressive dysplasia is present at birth and subluxation or dislocation has not yet developed, abnormal clinical signs may be absent or may be so subtle that early diagnosis is virtually impossible. There is no clinical finding that can universally be relied upon to detect all cases of CDH.

The incidence of CDH varies widely among races. It is approximately 1 in 60 in Caucasians when the condition is defined as detectable instability of the hip at birth. The incidence of complete dislocation at birth is about 1 in 500. For unknown reasons, blacks and Orientals are much less likely to develop CDH. Although many unstable neonatal hip joints will spontaneously become stable and develop normally, a substantial number will persist as unstable hips and become progressively deformed without treatment.

Two other orthopedic conditions have a recognized association with CDH. Approximately 10% to 20% of patients with congenital torticollis will show instability or dysplasia of the hip. In 1% of those infants with congenital foot deformities, most commonly metatarsus varus or calcaneovalgus, congenital dysplasia of the hip is found.

Etiology

The specific cause of CDH is unknown, but a multifactorial etiology is most likely. Three major factors in its causation are lack of acetabular depth, ligamentous laxity, and intrauterine breech positioning. During early formation, the fetal hip socket is quite deep and circumferentially contains the head of the femur. During continued growth, the acetabulum becomes increasingly shallow, until at birth acetabular depth is at its minimum. Thereafter, gradual deepening recurs, and the hip is normally well developed by the age of four years. The normal shallowness of the neonatal acetabulum predisposes it to instability.

The inherent ligamentous laxity and hypermobility of joints that occur in some families also predispose a child to development of CDH. In addition, the maternal hormone relaxin, which is present at term, is thought to influence the ligamentous integrity of the baby, particularly the female neonate. If the joints of a baby with inherent laxity are rendered even looser by hormonal influence, the hip joint has a greater risk of dislocating.

There is a statistical correlation between breech intrauterine positioning and the development of congenital hip dysplasia. Although the incidence of breech presentation in the general population is approximately 3%, 17% of all CDH occurs in breech-presentation babies. Seven per cent of breech-presentation female infants will have an unstable hip at birth, and 1 in 35 breech babies has established dislocation of the hip at birth. The hypothesis is that the breech-positioned individual has significant limitation of kicking and extension of the hip, and this allows for adaptive shortening of the iliopsoas muscle. Subsequently, when the newborn baby's hips are extended, the tightened muscle may lever the femoral head out of its shallow acetabulum.

Congenital dysplasia of the hip is more common in female infants, probably because of hormonally induced joint laxity and perhaps also because of the shape of the female pelvis. It is more common in the first born, which is considered by some to be caused by uterine tightness (which may disappear with subsequent pregnancies). It is also more common in children with a family history of CDH. Such environmental factors as ritualistic positioning of the neonate's lower extremities in hip extension and adduction may also increase the risk of instability or dislocation.

Pathology

Since a confluence of factors is necessary for hip dysplasia to occur, it is reasonable to expect a variable pathologic spectrum to result (Fig. 4–1). The severe end of the spectrum is the so-called "teratologic" or established intrauterine dislocation which, when detected at birth, is rarely reducible by closed means. The other end of the spectrum is the dislocatible hip, which is normally located

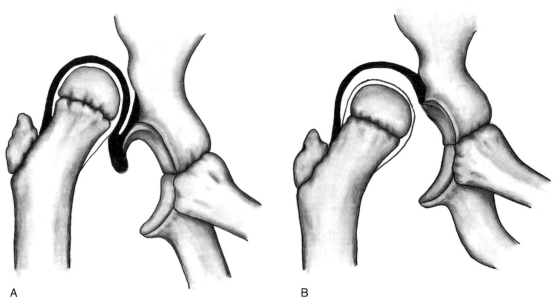

A   B

Figure 4–1. *A,* Congenital dislocation of the hip. The rim of the acetabulum is intact. *B,* Congenital subluxation of the hip. The acetabular rim has been eroded.

within the acetabulum but is easily dislocated by a maneuver of flexion, adduction, and posterior axial pressure on the thigh. This is known as Barlow's sign—a sudden acceleration as the hip leaves the acetabulum, followed by abrupt deceleration as the soft tissues become tight. The reverse of this is the Ortolani's sign, occurring when the dislocated hip suddenly accelerates as it glides over the rim and then abruptly decelerates as it seats into the depth of the acetabulum.

A different pathologic situation, the subluxation pattern, occurs when the acetabulum is deformed and assumes a shape much more oval than the normal hemisphere. This produces a shallower, elongated socket in which the unstable hip can slide up and down in degrees of instability ranging from barely detectable to obvious pistoning. In this situation, the acetabulum is more like a saucer than a cup.

The longer the hip joint develops abnormally, the more severe are the secondary adaptive changes. These include shortening of the musculotendinous structures that cross the hip joint, particularly the iliopsoas, rectus femoris, and hip adductor muscles, which may rapidly shorten to the extent that the hip cannot be reduced by closed means. If it can be reduced, however, it is only with markedly increased pressure on the femoral

head. A soft, cartilaginous, infantile femoral head that is compressed into the acetabulum under excessive pressure is at great risk of occlusion of its vascular channels, much as one would squeeze fluid from a sponge. In this case, the femoral head cannot be perfused with oxygenated blood, and avascular necrosis ensues, often with disastrous results. It is always essential that soft tissue contractures be overcome, either by preliminary traction or by surgical release, before attempts at reduction.

Other adaptive changes include failure of the empty acetabulum to deepen progressively with growth, flattening of the subluxed or dislocated femoral head as it is pressed against the wall of a flattened acetabulum or the pelvis, and increased valgus (increased neck-shaft angle) and anteversion (forward inclination) of the femoral neck. Changes also occur in the hip joint capsule, which surrounds the femoral head from its neck to the rim of the acetabulum like a sleeve. With dislocation, the capsule develops a stretched, waistlike, or hourglass constriction, so that even after traction has loosened the musculotendinous structures, the femoral head may not fit back through the isthmus of the capsule. This is analogous to attempting to push a button through a buttonhole that is too small (Fig. 4–2). This condition usually re-

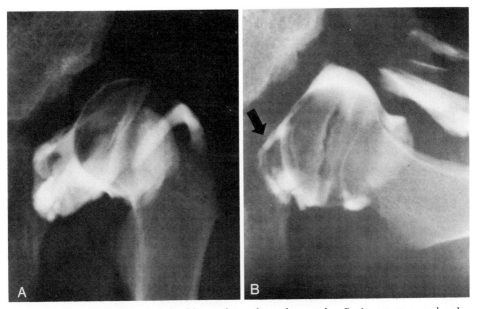

Figure 4–2. *A,* Congenital dislocation of the hip as shown by arthrography. *B,* An attempt at closed reduction following three weeks of traction failed because of interposed soft tissues *(arrow).* Open reduction was required.

sponds only to surgical division of both the hip capsule and the iliopsoas tendon in order to accomplish reduction.

Normal development of the hip may be impossible if adaptive changes have persisted long enough. Of primary importance in the management of congenital hip dysplasia, then, is early diagnosis, so that normal hip development (or as close to normal as possible) can occur.

Diagnosis in the Neonatal Period

Appreciating the variable pathologic factors involved in CDH, it is apparent that diagnosis in the neonatal period can be anything from quite simple and obvious to theoretically impossible. The most common diagnostic sign in the newborn is a hip that can be dislocated by Barlow's maneuver of flexion, adduction, and axial pressure in a posterior direction, or a hip that can be reduced by the Ortolani's maneuver, which essentially pulls the femoral head forward into the acetabulum by flexion, abduction, and lifting the femoral head anteriorly. Both these signs are easily missed in a baby who is crying and kicking. They may not be present at all in congenital subluxation (the saucer-shaped acetabulum) in which telescoping or pistoning of the hip is the significant finding. The condition may be detectable only with good relaxation of the hip musculature.

Another very reliable sign, significant at any age, is the apparently short femur (Fig. 4–3A). This is seen when the baby is lying supine and the hips and knees are flexed to 90 degrees. The level of the knees, i.e., the length of the thighs, should be equal. If one appears shorter than the other, the most likely reason is posterior subluxation or dislocation of the hip. This test goes by various names, including the Allis, Galeazzi, or Perkins sign, depending upon the position of the thighs, knees, and feet, but all are based upon the same anatomic condition. False-positive test results occur when there is true hypoplasia or shortening of the femur.

The most important and most reliable physical diagnostic maneuver for detecting subtle dysplasia in a neonatal hip is the assessment of the mobility triad. Since most fetuses develop in a knee-chest position, neonates normally have hip flexion contractures in the range of 20 to 40 degrees. Unless there

is frank breech positioning in utero, they have a lesser degree of knee flexion contracture as well (Fig. 4–3B). In addition, there is also a very mild adduction contracture (Fig. 4–3C). These contractures are known as the "mobility triad" and are normal and persistent throughout the first few months of life, before gradually being stretched out by the active infant. Normally, the hip flexion contracture is slightly greater than the knee flexion contracture, which is slightly greater than the hip adduction contracture. The importance of assessing the mobility triad is to detect asymmetry between the two sides in any or all of the three contractures. The most common finding is that when the hip is subluxed or dislocated posteriorly, it loses its stable fulcrum in the acetabulum. Proximal slipping occurs, thereby producing slack in the tight flexor muscles crossing the hip and causing loss of the normal flexion contracture on the involved side (Fig. 4–3D). The hamstring muscles are also slackened by posterior and superior displacement of the femoral head, and this causes disappearance of the knee flexion contracture on that side. The adduction contracture, however, becomes greater on the involved side because the adductor muscles are tightened by lateralization of the femoral head.

Other physical findings that often occur in the neonatal period are more subtle and less reliable, unless there is total dislocation of the hip. These include a fullness in the buttock as the femoral head is displaced posteriorly; a palpable hollow or depression in the anterior groin where the femoral head is normally located; significant widening of the perineum, seen in bilateral dislocation of the hip; and asymmetric posterior positioning of the greater trochanter. Asymmetric thigh skin folds, a frequently associated finding in CDH, also occur in approximately 30% of normal infants (Fig. 4–3E).

Radiographic study in the neonatal period is not necessarily diagnostic (Fig. 4–4). At this age, the femoral head is completely cartilaginous, and its ossific nucleus has not yet appeared. Not only mild degrees of hip dysplasia but also complete dislocation may be overlooked unless there is significant lateralization or proximal displacement of the femoral neck in relation to the acetabulum. Furthermore, an unstable hip may be reduced when the radiograph is taken and still be readily dislocatible.

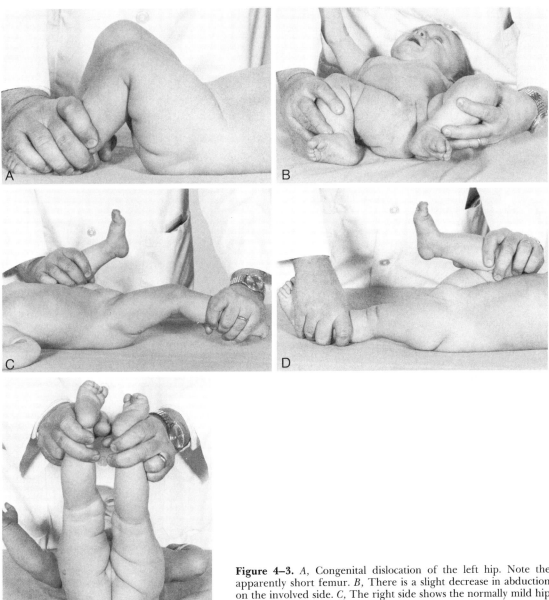

Figure 4–3. *A,* Congenital dislocation of the left hip. Note the apparently short femur. *B,* There is a slight decrease in abduction on the involved side. *C,* The right side shows the normally mild hip and knee flexion contractures of a neonate. *D,* The involved left side shows loss of the hip and knee flexion contractures. *E,* An apparently short left femur and asymmetric skin folds.

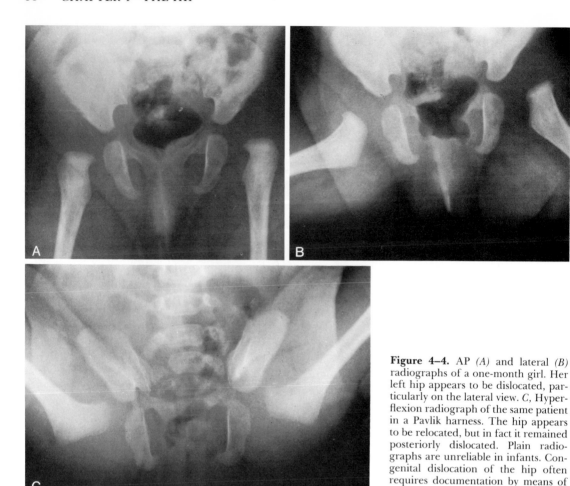

Figure 4–4. AP *(A)* and lateral *(B)* radiographs of a one-month girl. Her left hip appears to be dislocated, particularly on the lateral view. *C,* Hyperflexion radiograph of the same patient in a Pavlik harness. The hip appears to be relocated, but in fact it remained posteriorly dislocated. Plain radiographs are unreliable in infants. Congenital dislocation of the hip often requires documentation by means of hip arthrography.

Detection in Infancy

Although it is probable that most cases of CDH diagnosed between birth and the age of one year were detectable at birth, nevertheless some infants certainly exist who were either normal or so close to normal at birth that detection was not possible on clinical or radiographic examination. In either case, as the infant grows older, secondary adaptive changes occur, and the physical diagnostic picture changes. Usually by six weeks of age (and much earlier in most infants), the Ortolani's and Barlow's signs have disappeared. Either the hip is now not reducible or the acetabulum has become distorted so that the abrupt acceleration/deceleration phenomena do not occur. The femoral head may piston in a saucer-shaped acetabulum or may be dislocated, which makes closed reduction not possible.

In infancy, the most important diagnostic maneuver is again the assessment of the mobility triad. The usual findings in early infancy are loss of the normal hip flexion contracture and increase in the adduction contracture with loss of abduction on the involved side. The knee flexion contracture normally disappears in early infancy. Later in the first year of life, the normal hip flexion contracture may disappear. In this case, limitation of abduction is the most reliable component. The apparently short femur can also be present during this period and is a valuable diagnostic indicator. Other signs, such as buttock fullness or asymmetry, a hollow anterior groin, posterior positioning of the greater trochanter, and asymmetric thigh folds, become less noticeable as the infant grows older and may not be detectable at all. Nevertheless, it is vital to remember that the signs of mild CDH may be subtle and ex-

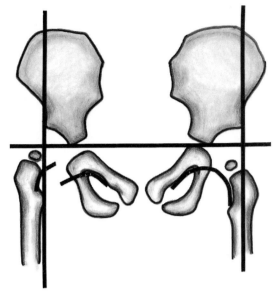

Figure 4–5. Congenital dislocation of the right hip. Quadrants are formed by drawing Hilgenreiner's line—a horizontal line through the triradiate cartilages—and Perkins' lines—vertical lines from the lateral edge of the acetabulae. A reduced femoral head should be in the lower inner quadrant, as seen on the patient's left. Shenton's line is a continuous arch from the medial femoral neck through the superior obturator foramen, as seen on the patient's left. The break in Shenton's line noted on the right is indicative of subluxation or dislocation.

of infants' hips be carried out at each well-baby check-up.

As infancy progresses, radiographic examination is diagnostic (Fig. 4–5). Such signs as lateral or proximal displacement of the femoral ossific nucleus, increased obliquity of the acetabular roof, a break in Shenton's line, and others are easily recognizable.

Detection in the Child Who is Walking

When the child begins walking, the most common diagnostic sign of hip dysplasia is an abnormal gait or limp. Although this is readily apparent in a completely dislocated hip, it can be extremely subtle with mild grades of dysplasia. It is therefore essential to study even a mild asymmetry or abnormality of gait in a preschool child by means of careful evaluation of the hips. In addition to gait disturbance, other findings in CDH after infancy include persistence of apparent shortening of the thigh and persistence of the hip adduction contracture. By walking age, the hip flexion and knee flexion contractures have normally disappeared.

Bilateral hip dislocation may be extremely difficult to detect, since the examination will be symmetric at any age. The most reliable signs are widening of the perineum, posterior displacement of the femoral heads, and positive results of Trendelenburg tests. Diagnosis by radiographic examination is precise in this age group, and even subtle signs are not difficult to detect (Fig. 4–6).

tremely difficult to detect during early infancy but will insidiously increase as the dysplasia progresses with growth. It is therefore essential that repeated careful examination

Figure 4–6. Congenital dislocation of the left hip. Note the hypoplasia of the femoral head and the dysplastic left acetabulum.

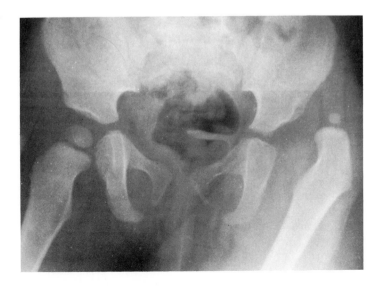

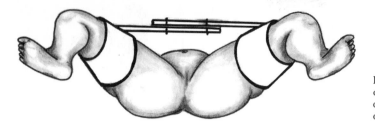

Figure 4–7. The proper position of abduction in a splint for congenital dislocation of the hip is no more than 60 degrees on each side.

Treatment

In the neonatal period, the majority of cases of hip joint instability or dislocation are easily reduced by accomplishing Ortolani's maneuver. With appropriate preventive splinting of the hip, reduction will be maintained, and the result will be the development of a normal joint. The position of immobilization is one of hyperflexion with no more than 60 degrees of abduction per hip (Fig. 4–7). This will avoid avascular necrosis in nearly all cases. Use of the Lorenz "frog" position of 90 degrees of abduction is absolutely contraindicated. This position compresses the major vascular supply to the femoral head. Great care must be taken to produce enough flexion and enough, but not excessive, abduction (45 to 60 degrees).

Because the degree of immobilization with triple diapering is very imprecise, a more appropriate splinting device, a plaster cast, or a Pavlik harness should be used. The best indication for triple diapering is the instance in which it is not possible to determine precisely whether hip disease is present. Still, one wishes to provide preventive treatment and to insure follow-up. Careful follow-up will detect cases of insidious subluxation with acetabular dysplasia, and these can be managed appropriately. If the neonatal hip is not easily reducible, then it is likely that secondary adaptive changes exist, and more complicated treatment is necessary.

In infancy, the simple preventive splinting or casting that was adequate treatment for most neonates is now inadequate because of secondary adaptive changes. Without careful evaluation and treatment of the patient, often including preliminary traction and arthrography, serious complications such as avascular necrosis, false reduction, redislocation, and progressive subluxation may occur (Fig. 4–8). Congenital dysplasia of the hip diag-

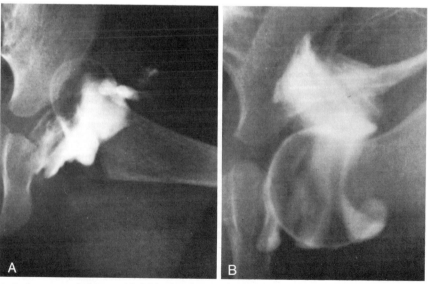

Figure 4–8. *A,* Arthrogram of dislocated left hip showing a spherical femoral head, which is displaced in the cephalad direction. *B,* Closed reduction shows perfect seating of the femoral head in the acetabulum. Note the homogeneous thin rim of dye surrounding the femoral head.

nosed after the neonatal period usually requires more complex orthopedic treatment. Some dysplasias in this period can be successfully treated with use of the Pavlik harness, but many require traction followed by reduction under arthrographic control and immobilization in plaster.

The management of older children with hip dysplasia is far more difficult than in younger age groups, and the achievement of a normal hip structure is less likely. After walking age, the majority will require open reduction, frequently combined with osteotomies of either the femur or the pelvis, or both.

It should be reemphasized that in many cases, the diagnosis of congenital dysplasia of the hip is not easy. It requires a high index of suspicion and persistence on the part of the examiner. Even then, skilled physicians will occasionally miss subtle cases. An abnormality in the physical findings of the neonate, infant, or older child must be satisfactorily explained by means of further evaluation and radiographic study. Plain radiographs are occasionally misleading in the first three months of life and should not be accepted as absolute evidence of a normal hip during this period. An adequate program for the detection of congenital hip dysplasia includes thorough newborn examinations and preventive treatment when indicated, careful reexamination during infancy at each well-baby check-up, and particular attention to any gait abnormality in an ambulatory child.

CONGENITAL ANOMALIES OF THE HIP AND FEMUR

Developmental anomalies of the femur include coxa vara, congenital short femur, and proximal focal femoral deficiency.

Coxa Vara

In the normal infant's proximal femur, the neck-shaft angle measures in the range of 140 to 155 degrees. When measured from the horizontal axis, the growth plate makes an angle of 20 to 30 degrees. Generically, "coxa vara" is a term that can be applied to any condition in which the neck-shaft angle is abnormally acute. This can result from known pathologic entities such as fibrous dysplasia, rickets, osteogenesis imperfecta,

and other conditions in which bone strength is impaired. It is also common in bone dysplasias and certain dwarfing conditions.

Idiopathic or developmental coxa vara is usually not associated with other conditions, with the exception of occasional shortening of the femur. The condition is not detectable at birth and most often is noted only after the child has been walking several months. It presents either as a limp or as a waddling type of gait, depending upon whether it is unilateral or bilateral. Bilateral involvement occurs about one third of the time, with these patients also being short in stature. On clinical examination, hip range of motion is limited, the extent of limitation depending upon the severity of the condition. Loss of abduction and internal rotation is the rule, and compensatory genu valgum and hyperlordosis are often seen (Fig. 4–9). The cause of developmental coxa vara is unknown, but it can be inherited as an autosomal dominant trait.

Radiographs of coxa vara show a decrease in the neck-shaft angle; shortening of the femoral neck; a more-vertical-than-normal angle of the growth plate; and new bone formation along the medial femoral neck, probably in an attempt to buttress the progressive varus (Fig. 4–10). This new bone frequently has a triangular appearance.

If left untreated, the limp and loss of motion are progressive; premature fusion of the growth plate with further shortening occurs; and premature degenerative arthritis is often seen. Appropriate treatment consists of performance of a valgus osteotomy. Great care must be taken to restore precisely the angle of the growth plate to less than 30 degrees but not to increase the length of the bone, since this may result in increased pressure on the femoral head and subsequent avascular necrosis.

Congenital Short Femur

When recognized at birth, this condition may be mistaken for congenital dislocation of the hip because of the unequal lengths of the thighs. Careful clinical examination reveals shortening of the involved femur when compared with that on the opposite side. On radiographic examination, the hip joint is normal, and the femur, besides being short, may have increased anterior or lateral bowing, or both. Coxa vara may also be present.

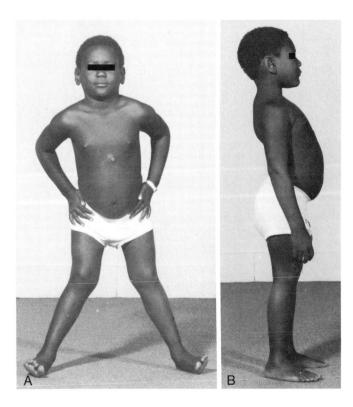

Figure 4–9. *A,* Bilateral congenital coxa vara. A striking finding is the severe compensatory genu valgum. *B,* The coxa vara is associated with hyperlordosis in the lumbar spine secondary to anterior tilting of the pelvis.

The management of this condition begins with determining the difference in length as a percentage of the length of the normal femur. This percentage difference will remain constant in the majority of cases, so that the appropriate time for leg length equalization can be calculated. Once the discrepancy exceeds two centimeters in the growing child, correction should be obtained with use of a shoe lift. If the adult discrepancy is projected to be more than two centimeters, distal femoral epiphyseodesis is indicated on the long side at the appropriate age. If more than four centimeters' difference is anticipated, femoral lengthening may be the best solution.

Proximal Focal Femoral Deficiency

Proximal focal femoral deficiency (PFFD) describes a spectrum of abnormalities occurring in the proximal portion of the femur, ranging from slight hypoplasia to complete absence of the upper end of the bone. The distal half of the femur is usually normal but may be hypoplastic. Nearly half the cases also have fibular hemimelia. The clinical presentation of PFFD consists of shortening of the thigh with associated external rotation and flexion contractures at the hip (Fig. 4–11). Bilaterality is uncommon. One should also look for other anomalies in both the musculoskeletal and other systems.

As with other conditions that present as a spectrum of disorders, several classifications of this deformity have been proposed. Most

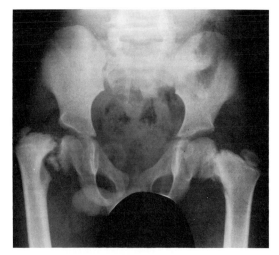

Figure 4–10. Bilateral infantile coxa vara.

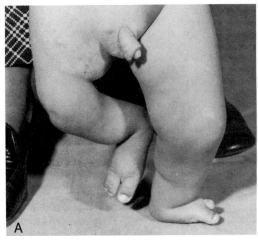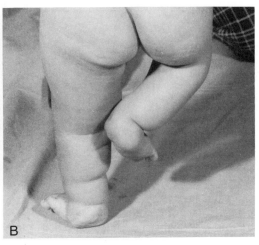

Figure 4–11. *A,* Proximal focal femoral deficiency of the right femur. Note the marked shortening of the thigh and the absence of lateral foot rays bilaterally. This patient had associated bilateral fibular hemimelia. *B,* A posterior view of the same patient.

of them are based upon whether the femoral head is present and, if so, whether there is continuity between the head and the shaft of the femur. Because treatment is based on the severity of involvement, it is important to determine early in the patient's life whether the femoral head is present. Since it may be cartilaginous in the infantile period, arthrography or computerized tomography may be very helpful (Fig. 4–12). Function is much better if there is a femoral head and if the head is in continuity with the femoral shaft. Individuals with discontinuity or tenuous continuity may be considered for bone grafting. Most patients who have unilateral PFFD and severe shortening of the lower limb ultimately undergo amputation of the foot and fusion of the knee and are fitted with a

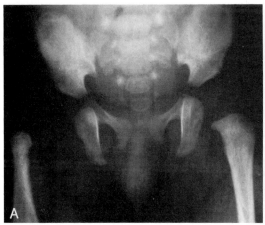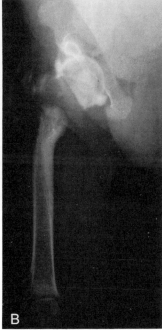

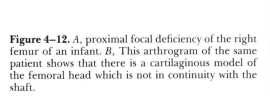

Figure 4–12. *A,* proximal focal deficiency of the right femur of an infant. *B,* This arthrogram of the same patient shows that there is a cartilaginous model of the femoral head which is not in continuity with the shaft.

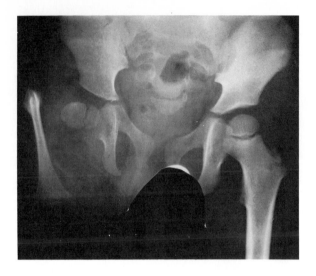

Figure 4–13. Proximal focal deficiency of the right femur. Note the ossified femoral head and neck, which is discontinuous with the shaft and in marked varus.

prosthesis as a long, above-knee amputee (Fig. 4–13). In such cases, those with a stable hip will function much better than those amputees with no proximal femur and significant hip instability. The treatment strategy for bilateral cases is completely different. The majority of these are best left untreated.

INFECTION IN OR AROUND THE HIP JOINT

Septic Arthritis

In children, an infection in any major joint, but particularly in the hip, usually has major implications for subsequent function. Interruption of the blood supply or direct invasion of the cartilage and bone can produce substantial damage and disruption of future growth. Long-term effects may include bone shortening, angular deformity, joint surface irregularities, stiffness, and early degenerative changes.

Approximately two thirds of all cases of septic arthritis occur before the age of three. It is slightly more common in males. About 80% of the cases involve joints of the lower extremity, the hip being the most commonly involved site. The most common causative organism after the age of two years is *Staphylococcus aureus*. In infancy, *Haemophilus influenzae* type B is most common.

In children, the mechanism of onset is either direct extension of osteomyelitis from the proximal metaphysis of the femur into the hip joint, or hematogenous dissemination of organisms via the blood supply of the synovial membrane. Once the infection becomes established, a direct attack by synovial collagenase causes cartilage destruction. Lysosomal enzymes from the white blood cells can also destroy cartilage matrix, exposing collagen fibers which are then mechanically eroded.

The clinical presentation of septic arthritis is a warm, painful, tender joint with reflex muscle spasm and limited motion. Unfortunately, by the time these signs are evident, substantial damage may already have occurred. A high index of suspicion with the infant who has minimal early symptoms and signs, including irritability and poor feeding, is essential.

The most important diagnostic procedure is aspiration of purulent fluid from the joint. This may require general anesthesia and arthrography. If joint sepsis is suspected and no fluid is obtained upon aspiration, then the joint should be irrigated with saline and the resulting aspirant cultured. Positive results of joint and blood cultures confirm the diagnosis. Laboratory studies show increase in the sedimentation rate with a normal or only slightly increased white blood cell count. Anemia is common. Early radiographic changes are capsular distention and widening of the hip joint space. As the process evolves, increased pressure inside the joint causes thrombosis of the nutrient vessels to the femoral capital epiphysis. If treatment is delayed, the results will be poor (Fig. 4–14).

The treatment of septic arthritis of the hip is immediate surgical drainage and antibiotic therapy. The surgical preference is an anterior or posterior exposure of the hip joint; irrigation of necrotic debris, the fibrin clot, and purulent material; and insertion of a drain. The wound is left open. The patient is then placed in a spica cast with a window over the hip and kept in the appropriate position for dependent drainage. A good reason for anterior drainage is that the critical blood supply to the immature femoral head comes primarily through the posterior part of the joint, and the anterior approach avoids possible disruption of this blood supply.

Administration of intravenous antibiotics is started preoperatively. The choice of antibiotic is influenced by the results of the smear, the most likely organism based on the patient's age, and current data regarding prevalent organisms and infections in the community. When the culture results become available, a change of drug may be necessary. When the infection is under control and drainage has essentially ceased, range of motion exercises are begun. Oral antibiotics are given until the sedimentation rate has returned to normal.

It is worthwhile to emphasize that systemic antibiotic levels in septic joint fluids equal or exceed serum levels, and intra-articular antibiotic injections are unnecessary and probably contraindicated. The fibrin clot and debris in the joint will trap organisms and cannot be adequately aspirated from the hip,

no matter what size the needle. Arthrotomy of a septic major joint is essential and is a surgical emergency. It is necessary to assure adequate drainage and give the maximum chance to avoid permanent damage to the joint.

Osteomyelitis

Osteomyelitis is very much a problem of pediatric practice, since 85% of this disease occurs in patients younger than 16 years of age. The ratio of male to female involvement is approximately four to one. The portal of entry in children is almost always hematogenous, except in cases of contaminated open wounds and rare instances of local extension from a nearby infected focus. The majority of cases at any age are caused by *Staphylococcus aureus*.

The pathology of osteomyelitis of the proximal femur depends upon the vascular anatomy, which in turn is related to the age of the child. At any age, however, the infection usually begins in the metaphyseal region. During the first 12 to 18 months of life, the growth plate is traversed by vascular channels of communication between the epiphysis and the metaphysis. This means that there is little resistance to the extension of infection across the physis in the proximal femur. For this reason, osteomyelitis in the infantile period can rapidly destroy the femoral head, and it

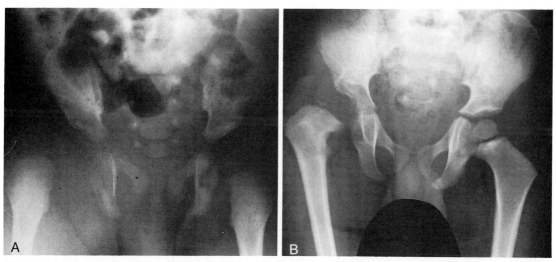

Figure 4–14. *A,* Septic arthritis of the right hip with lateralization of the proximal femur and marked soft tissue swelling. *B,* Four years later, there is destruction of the femoral head, deformity of the proximal femur, and severe subluxation of the hip.

often extends into the hip joint to become septic arthritis. After infancy, the growth plate acts as a barrier, since the vascular channels traversing it have dropped out. Infections that are initially localized to the metaphyseal region may reach the hip joint by erosion through the thinned metaphyseal cortex, which is intracapsular. The metaphyseal region of a bone is the most common site of onset of osteomyelitis because the arteriolar loops feed into a relatively large venous capillary bed, where blood flow is slow and oxygen tension is low. This predisposes the area to the seeding of pathogenic bacteria.

The diagnostic picture of osteomyelitis of the proximal femur is quite variable, depending upon the age of the patient. In the infant, fever and signs of systemic toxicity are usually absent, and the most common signs are irritability, poor feeding, localized limb edema, and pseudoparalysis (muscle guarding and unwillingness to move the affected limb). In the older child, signs of sepsis are the rule. Localized signs of inflammation are present, and protective reflex myospasm is seen. Clearly, the time it takes to examine the motion of a child's hip gently and to compare it with that of the other side may be well worthwhile if the cause of a child's lethargy, irritability, poor feeding, or fever is osteomyelitis of the proximal femur. Whenever there is *any* question of possible septic arthritis or osteomyelitis, the hip joint *must* be aspirated.

The diagnosis of osteomyelitis by radiographic examination depends upon the stage of the pathologic process. The first sign is loss of soft tissue planes, usually within the first three to five days following the onset of the infection. There may be some early hip joint widening, caused by a "sympathetic effusion" at this time. Following this, some mottling of bone density is seen, usually occurring in the first 7 to 12 days. At this time, if the infection has eroded into the hip joint, substantial widening of the joint space is seen. Later in the course of osteomyelitis, new bone formation and further central bony destruction continue. The late radiographic findings show destruction of the proximal femur.

The diagnosis of proximal femoral osteomyelitis by means of laboratory tests involves isolation of the causative organism, either by obtaining a blood culture or by direct aspiration from the femoral neck with performance of a smear and culture. Aspiration can quickly be accomplished under fluoroscopic control with the patient under general anesthesia. The erythrocyte sedimentation rate is increased, and white blood cell counts are usually either normal or slightly increased with a leftward shift. A general search of other organ systems for a primary site of infection and obtaining appropriate cultures are also essential.

The treatment of acute osteomyelitis begins with immediate institution of intravenous antibiotic therapy in adequate dosages, based on the most likely causative organism. The drug should be started as soon as blood and local cultures have been obtained. The length of time that the intravenous route is used depends upon the organism, the drug, and the patient's response. Antibiotics should be continued by either intravenous or oral administration until the sedimentation rate has returned to normal. If the oral route is selected, it is important to monitor peak and trough antibiotic concentrations in the serum. This usually requires inpatient care to assure compliance. During the acute phase of the infection, bed rest, immobilization, analgesics, and hydration are important and, if indicated, surgical decompression. The most common reason for surgical decompression of acute osteomyelitis is to drain suspected pus under pressure; that is, when a lytic lesion is seen in the proximal femur. This is usually best accomplished through either an anterior or a lateral approach to avoid damage to the posterior epiphyseal vessels. Another indication for surgical treatment is to obtain a diagnosis when other attempts have failed. The surgical treatment includes cutting a small window in the periosteum and bony cortex, performing a curettage of material for culture, and then allowing open drainage. Rapid granulation and healing of the wound is the rule once the infection is under control.

Chronic osteomyelitis of the proximal femur is usually seen in association with profound destruction of the femoral head and neck. Fortunately, it is extremely rare, but when present aggressive surgical treatment is required to eradicate the infection. Profound shortening of the limb will almost always result. The options for surgical reconstruction and salvage in such cases are never very satisfactory.

In summary, it is difficult to overstate the importance of early diagnosis and prompt, aggressive surgical and antibiotic treatment for infections of the hip and proximal femur. Therapeutic efforts are a race against time if one is to prevent permanent damage to the growth plate and to the femoral head and neck, along with the subsequent possibility of angular and linear deformity, pathologic fracture, chronic osteomyelitis, pain, stiffness, and profound interference with function.

LEGG-PERTHES DISEASE (LEGG-CALVÉ-PERTHES DISEASE)

Legg-Perthes disease is avascular necrosis of the femoral head. It was first described during the period from 1908 to 1910 by Arthur T. Legg of Boston, Jacques Calvé of France, and Georg Perthes of Germany. The disease has an incidence of approximately 1 in 1500, with males outnumbering females by a ratio of about six to one. The right and left hips are approximately equally affected, and bilateral cases occur at least 15% of the time. If one child is involved, the risk of a sibling developing the condition increases from 1 in 1500 to 1 in 25. Legg-Perthes disease is seen from three to 12 years of age, with a peak at the age of six years. More than 50% of the cases occur between the ages of five and seven.

Etiology

The specific cause of the avascular necrosis in Legg-Perthes disease is unknown, but in some cases there may be either a genetic predisposition to or an association with, or both, trauma, recurrent synovitis, and a retarded bone age. Almost 90% of the patients have retardation of their skeletal age, as determined by the method of Greulich and Pyle. Transient synovitis may have an effect on the onset of this condition, possibly by increasing intra-articular pressure in the hip joint or by interfering with the vascular supply to the femoral head. It has been documented that in some cases, multiple episodes of avascular insult to the femoral head have occurred.

Pathology

Legg-Perthes disease goes through five sequential stages: prenecrosis, necrosis, revascularization, reossification, and remodeling.

During the prenecrosis stage, there is vascular shutdown, which may be related to trauma to the arterial supply, hypercoagulability and thrombosis, microemboli, increased intra-articular pressure, or positional arterial compression. Venous occlusion may also be a primary factor.

During the necrosis stage, the involved bone of the femoral epiphysis, and sometimes the metaphysis, is dead. Tensile strength of the bone is reduced, and micro- or macrofractures occur in the femoral head. The involved bone ceases to grow, and in more severe cases, cyst formation occurs. The infarct may involve only a small segment of the femoral head or it may include the entire head, physis, and metaphysis as well. The necrosis stage lasts three to six months. A crescent-shaped subchondral fracture is often seen in this stage (Fig. 4–15).

The revascularization stage is initiated as dead bone is resorbed and replaced with vascularized granulation tissue. During this stage, deformity may occur with anterior and lateral extrusion of the "softened" femoral head from the acetabulum (Fig. 4–16). True hypertrophy of the femoral head occurs owing to the unabated growth of preosseous cartilage. Secondary acetabular flattening also occurs. This stage usually lasts 6 to 12 months.

The reossification stage occurs when the molded and deformed femoral head gradually reossifies (Fig. 4–17). Reossification takes place from the periphery to the center, and it may take 18 months to 3 years to complete.

The final stage is remodeling, during which there may be gradual but often minimal improvement in the congruity of the hip joint (Fig. 4–18). The natural history of Legg-Perthes disease is a protracted course, lasting at least one to three years. The femoral head always revascularizes but is almost always deformed. In spite of this, most patients have a good long-term prognosis and will not experience significant pain or loss of motion. Most will not require reconstructive hip arthroplasty.

Diagnosis

The diagnosis of Legg-Perthes disease is based upon the clinical picture, radiographic examination, and, if needed, technetium bone scanning (Fig. 4–19). The clinical picture includes a constant or transient limp, or

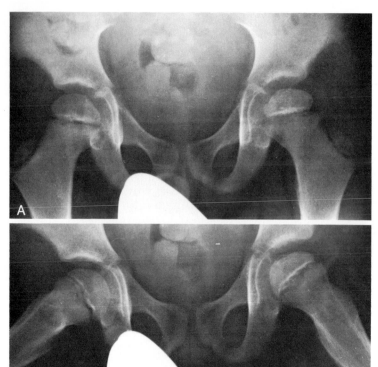

Figure 4–15. *A*, Legg-Perthes disease of the left hip. Note the slightly flattened femoral head. A small subchondral fracture line is visible in the upper center of the head. There is also slight widening of the medial joint–cartilage space. *B*, The lateral view demonstrates the subchondral fracture with mild flattening in the anterolateral quadrant of the femoral head. One would anticipate slightly greater than 50% avascularity of the femoral head.

Figure 4–16. Legg-Perthes disease of the right hip. Note involvement of the entire femoral head and the metaphysis. There is also calcification, which appears lateral to the femoral epiphysis but in fact represents subluxation.

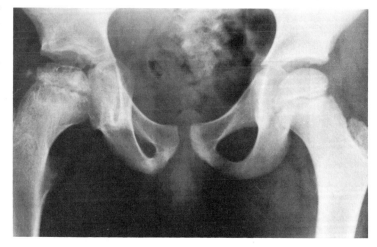

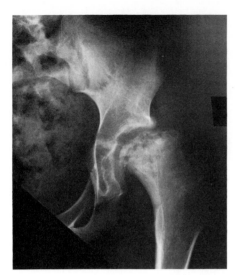

Figure 4–17. Severe deformity of the left hip as a result of untreated Legg-Perthes disease with total femoral head involvement. The femoral head is reossifying.

Widening of the medial joint space is apparent because of this same failure of growth. This is often associated with some degree of loss of bone density in the metaphysis. Later signs include a crescent-shaped subchondral fracture in the femoral head, shortening of the femoral neck (coxa breva), and flattening (coxa plana) and ultimately enlargement (coxa magna) of the femoral head. Assessment of the extent of the subchondral fracture allows a satisfactory diagnosis to be made. Before its appearance, however, a bone scan will be of great value (Fig. 4–21). Bone scan findings confirm the diagnosis and provide an excellent means of quantifying the extent of avascularity and, therefore, of determining the prognosis and guiding treatment. As a rule of thumb, the lesser the amount of avascular bone and the younger the child at the onset of disease, the better the prognosis, although there is always some residual deformity of the hip seen on radiographs. The key factor in a good prognosis is congruity between femoral head and acetabulum after remodeling.

some other gait abnormality; pain, which may be referred to the anterior thigh or may be present in the anterior or lateral hip area; loss of hip motion, particularly rotation and abduction; atrophy of the thigh and buttock muscles; tenderness to palpation over the hip joint, which signifies synovitis; and usually retardation of the skeletal age.

Radiographic findings depend upon the stage of the process (Fig. 4–20). The earliest sign is failure of the epiphysis to grow, best demonstrated on the lateral view by comparing the involved and the uninvolved hip.

Treatment

The goals of treatment in Legg-Perthes disease are to prevent subluxation, to preserve as much as possible the sphericity of the femoral head, and to maintain good muscle function to allow for a normal gait. Early treatment consists of clearing up muscle spasm and synovitis by means of bed rest, often combined with Russell's or Buck's skin

Figure 4–18. This patient had "silent" Legg-Perthes disease at age six with resultant early closure of the proximal growth plate. Note the marked shortening of the femoral neck with relative proximal extension of the greater trochanter, producing passive insufficiency in the hip abductor muscles. The hip joint was relatively congruous, and leg function was good. She required epiphysiodesis of the left distal femur to equalize limb lengths.

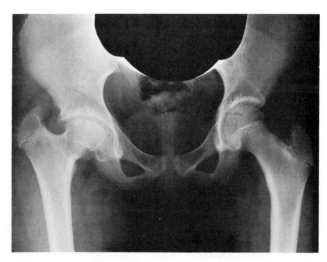

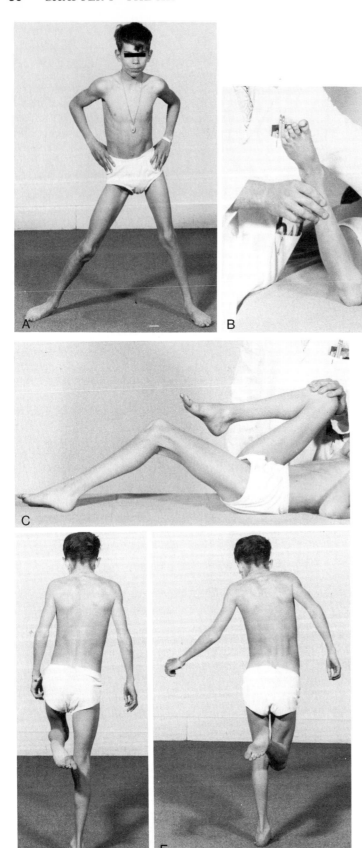

Figure 4–19. *A*, Legg-Perthes disease of the left hip. Note the limitation of abduction and the atrophy of the left thigh. *B*, Loss of internal rotation on the involved side. *C*, The involved side has a significant hip flexion contracture. *D*, A normal response to the Trendelenburg test. When the patient is standing on the noninvolved leg, the abductor muscles are able to maintain balance by elevating the contralateral pelvis. *E*, A Trendelenburg sign with positive results on the involved side. Because of pain and weakness, the abductors are unable to maintain pelvic balance, and the patient must compensate by leaning toward the left.

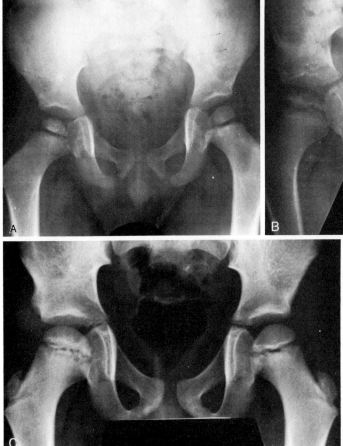
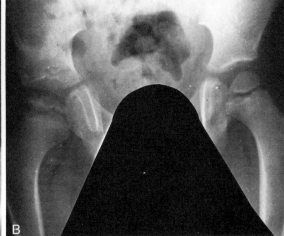
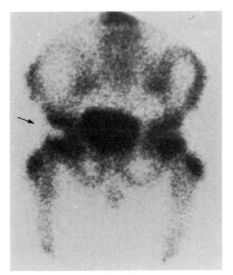

Figure 4–20. *A*, Early Legg-Perthes disease of the right hip. Note the failure of the epiphyseal nucleus to grow and the widening of the medial joint space. *B*, The hip is now in the stage of bony resorption. An innominate osteotomy has been performed to maintain containment of the femoral head. *C*, The long-term result is a well-contained, congruous femoral head.

Figure 4–21. A technetium bone scan showing avascularity consistent with Legg-Perthes disease of the right hip.

traction. Once the patient is comfortable and has an improved range of motion, the definitive treatment can begin.

Observation only is appropriate for almost all cases with minimal involvement of the femoral head (less than 50%), regardless of age. A better result will be achieved with hips that have not yet reossified and that have greater than 50% involvement if they are treated by some means that achieves containment of the femoral head within the acetabulum. This is accomplished by abduction and can be done by using an abduction orthosis (Fig. 4–22). Alternatively, surgical means can be used, either by redirecting the acetabulum laterally over the femoral head or by performing a varus osteotomy of the proximal femur (Fig. 4–23). There is good evidence that in patients with more severe grades of involvement, containment of the femoral head produces a more congruous,

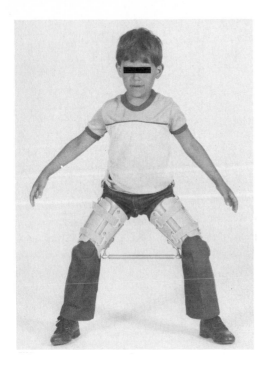

Figure 4–22. A six-year-old boy with Legg-Perthes disease of the right hip. He is being treated with the Atlanta Scottish Rite abduction orthosis, which provides for abduction and flexion. It is widely used in the nonoperative treatment of Legg-Perthes disease.

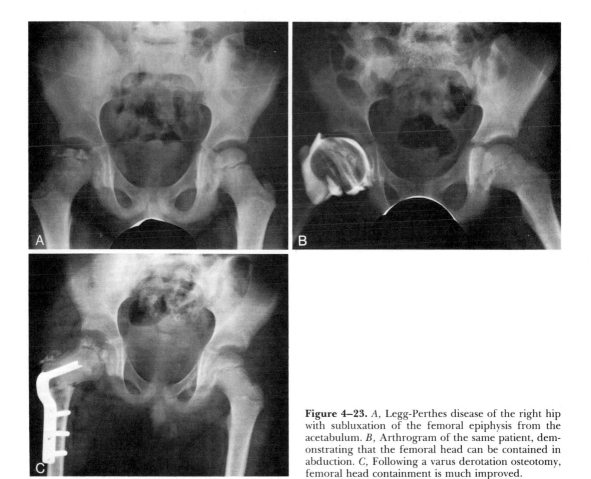

Figure 4–23. *A*, Legg-Perthes disease of the right hip with subluxation of the femoral epiphysis from the acetabulum. *B*, Arthrogram of the same patient, demonstrating that the femoral head can be contained in abduction. *C*, Following a varus derotation osteotomy, femoral head containment is much improved.

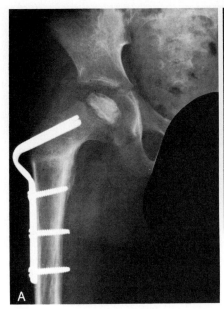
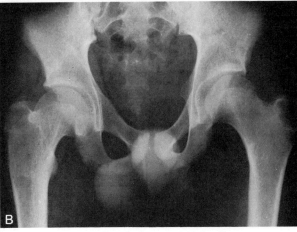

Figure 4–24. *A,* Total involvement of the right femoral capital epiphysis in Legg-Perthes disease after treatment with a varus derotation osteotomy. *B,* Nine years later, the result is excellent.

better result than does no treatment. The younger the patient, the more rapid the course of the disease and, therefore, the more likely one is to select an orthosis. For an older patient, for example a nine-year-old child with severe involvement, many believe that the conservative treatment is a surgical procedure rather than having the child spend two to three years in a cumbersome orthosis.

Occasionally, patients with Legg-Perthes disease are first seen during the stage of reossification and already have a flattened, subluxated femoral head. In such cases, it is best to wait until complete healing and remodeling have occurred. Then such salvage procedures as cheilectomy, valgus osteotomy, or Chiari osteotomy may be of value.

The ultimate outcome of Legg-Perthes disease is often better than one would expect from the radiographic changes (Fig. 4–24). The best results occur in hips that have the best congruity of the opposing joint surfaces, regardless of the flattening. Other good prognostic signs are lack of lateralization or extrusion, good range of motion, and onset of the disease at an early age.

SLIPPED CAPITAL FEMORAL EPIPHYSIS

Slipped capital femoral epiphysis (SCFE) may develop either as an abrupt or as a gradual displacement of the femoral head from the femoral neck. The slipping occurs through the growth plate. The term is something of a misnomer, since the head is actually contained in the acetabulum by the acetabular contour; the neck displaces, usually anteriorly and slightly superiorly. The incidence of SCFE is approximately 1 per 50,000. It occurs two to three times more commonly in males than in females, and occurs more often in blacks than in Caucasians. It almost always occurs during preadolescence or adolescence. The likelihood of occurrence of bilateral slipped epiphyses is 25% to 50% in most studies.

Etiology

Because a single specific causative agent has not been identified, it is probable that most patients develop this condition from a confluence of factors. These may include the fact that the physis is weaker during the adolescent growth spurt; trauma (the rate of occurrence is higher in the spring and summer months); perhaps an inflammatory or autoimmune process; hormonal factors, particularly in those conditions affecting growth hormone or changes in estrogen or testosterone balance; an intrinsic defect in the growth plate; and increased body mass and obesity. Approximately 50% of the patients are obese, and many are at greater than the ninetieth percentile in height. Finally, genetic factors may play a role, since approximately 4% of the patients with SCFE have a family history of this condition.

Signs and Symptoms

Ten to 20% of cases seem to occur as an acute, sudden event, although with careful questioning previous mild symptoms may often be discovered. An acute slip causes painful weight bearing. The pain is usually localized to the anterior and lateral groin, thigh, or knee, or to a combination of the three. Physical examination shows painful motion in most ranges, with marked limitation of internal rotation and abduction. The extremity may appear slightly shortened. Flexing the involved hip produces concomitant external rotation, and this is pathognomonic for a slipped epiphysis (Fig. 4–25). More subtle cases generally will have a history of mild intermittent pain and limping, occasionally with associated weakness of the involved lower extremity. Symptoms may be present for an extended period of time, even for years in some cases. It is important to note, however, that some slips are asymptomatic or "silent."

Diagnosis

All patients in the preadolescent or adolescent period with any symptoms or signs re-

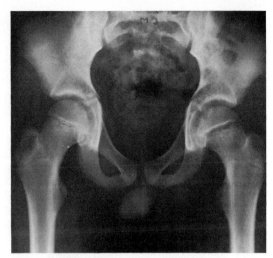

Figure 4–26. AP view of the pelvis showing widening of the growth plate of the proximal left femur—an early sign of a slipped capital femoral epiphysis.

ferable to the hips should be suspected of having a slip of the capital femoral epiphysis until proven otherwise. The earliest radiographic signs of subtle slips are widening of the growth plate and mild osteopenia of the proximal femur when compared with the uninvolved side, but usually with little or no displacement of the epiphysis in either the anteroposterior (AP) or lateral view (Fig. 4–26). Biplanar views are essential to the diagnosis of this condition, since many slips are almost purely posterior and cannot be easily detected on an AP view. It should be remembered that forced flexion to obtain a "frog lateral" radiograph has the potential for increasing the displacement of the slip. Therefore, a true cross-table lateral view should be obtained for suspected cases. With more significant slipping, the radiographs show loss of the normal continuity between the head and neck of the femur (Fig. 4–27). In chronic slips, remodeling changes are seen along the superior and anterior femoral neck.

Clinical Significance

The significance of a slipped epiphysis includes the potential for further slipping, the potential for interference with normal gait, the potential for interruption of the vascular or nutritional supply to the bone and cartilage of the hip joint, and the potential for

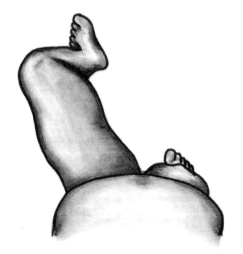

Figure 4–25. Slipped capital femoral epiphysis of the left hip. As the hip is flexed, the leg goes into external rotation and abduction.

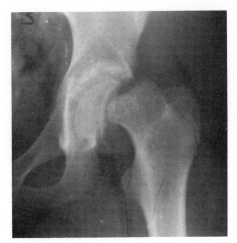

Figure 4–27. A severe inferior slip of the capital femoral epiphysis.

the development of premature degenerative arthritis of the hip. Further slipping carries substantial risk. The femoral head, which becomes dissociated from its metaphysis, often loses its blood supply and undergoes avascular necrosis. This leads to a stiff, painful hip, a disaster for an adolescent. Any hip with an identified slip, either acute or chronic, must be considered at risk for further slipping and treated as a situation of extreme urgency. The patient should not be allowed to walk but should be placed in a recumbent or sitting position and transported directly to qualified orthopedic care.

Avascular necrosis can occur as the result of the slip itself or as the result of overzealous manipulation in the reduction or surgical treatment of the slip. With avascular necrosis, there is ultimately collapse, either total or partial, of the femoral head. Chondrolysis is a condition in which the cartilage of the femoral head degenerates, producing joint narrowing, stiffness, contracture, pain, and limping. It may be idiopathic in origin, but it has also been associated with severe slips and with trauma to the articular surface experienced during therapeutic efforts.

The person who has had a slipped capital femoral epiphysis has a higher than normal risk of developing degenerative arthritis. The long-term prognosis depends upon the amount of displacement, the more severe slips having a greater likelihood of degenerating in later life.

A deformed proximal femur with restricted abduction and internal rotation has a negative effect on the normal gait cycle. It causes a noticeable limp, which translates into greater energy requirements during walking. The center of gravity must undergo greater displacement with each cycle of gait, and this predisposes the patient to greater fatigability.

Treatment

The objectives of treatment of SCFE are to prevent further slipping and to gain gentle correction, if possible, while minimizing the risk of avascular necrosis or chondrolysis. If the slip is minimal, the range of motion is not much altered, and simple in situ fixation of the slip by insertion of multiple pins or by open-bone-graft epiphyseodesis is the treatment of choice (Figs. 4–28 and 4–29). An alternative is prolonged hip immobilization in a spica cast. An acute slip may respond to gentle reduction by means of traction or gentle manipulation and in situ pinning. Many acute slips are, in reality, superimposed upon chronic slips. In these cases, an attempt to gain anatomic reduction will result in avascular necrosis. A substantial slip of chronic duration cannot be reduced. This requires an osteotomy and removal of a biplanar

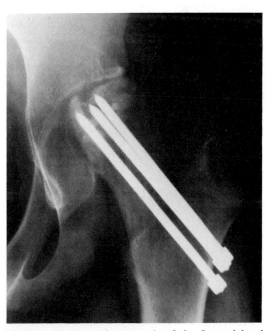

Figure 4–28. Avascular necrosis of the femoral head with fragmentation and collapse following pinning of a slipped capital femoral epiphysis.

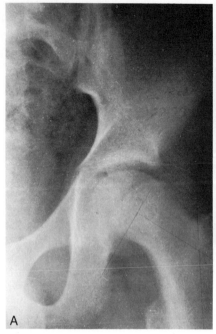

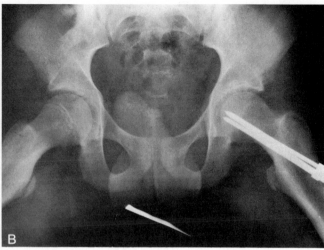

Figure 4–29. *A*, Slipped capital femoral epiphysis of the left hip. *B*, Following gentle closed reduction and pinning, further slipping has been prevented. The physis has closed.

wedge of bone, followed by internal fixation, to restore more normal gait mechanics and weight-bearing forces in the femoral head (Fig. 4–30).

The most important considerations regarding SCFE are to have a high index of suspicion for this problem in any preadolescent or adolescent with a limp or with hip, thigh, or knee pain, and to confirm or rule out the diagnosis immediately with use of appropriate biplanar radiographs. Once the diagnosis has been made, even a chronic slip is at risk of progressing, and the patient should be promptly referred for orthopedic treatment without being allowed to walk or bear weight on the involved side.

HIP PAIN IN CHILDREN AND ADOLESCENTS

"Hip pain" is a generic term used to describe discomfort referable to the sensory innervation provided by the obturator or femoral nerves, or both. It can be produced by any type of lesion in the region of the hip joint: in its capsule and synovial lining, in the bone of the pelvis or proximal femur, or in the muscles, nerves, and vascular structures in the region of the hip, buttock, groin, or pelvis. Regardless of cause, the hip pain is usually localized to the region of the anterior groin, of the greater trochanter, or of the anterolateral thigh down to the knee (Fig. 4–31). It is imperative that hip pain be evaluated thoroughly and its cause determined, since many of the causes urgently need treatment and may carry a bad prognosis.

The differential diagnosis of hip pain includes tumors of the pelvis, spine, or proximal femur; infections, particularly of the hip

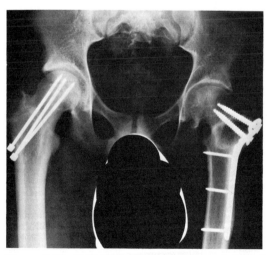

Figure 4–30. A 14-year-old boy with bilateral slipped capital femoral epiphysis. In situ pinning was done on the right hip and a Southwick osteotomy on the left. The results were good on both hips.

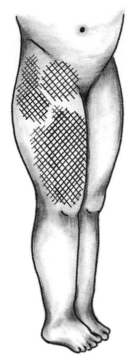

Figure 4–31. The distribution of referred pain from hip disease in children.

joint and proximal femur (but pelvic and intervertebral disc space infections can also present with hip pain); slipped capital femoral epiphysis, on either a chronic or an acute traumatic basis; Legg-Perthes disease; and various metabolic conditions such as juvenile rheumatoid arthritis or early osteoarthritis. Finally, a common cause of hip pain in children is synovitis, which is often a diagnosis of exclusion.

HIP PAIN CAUSED BY SYNOVITIS

Synovitis, also known as "observation hip," toxic synovitis, or "irritable hip," is not a rare phenomenon. It occurs more commonly in males and is usually seen after the age of two years but before skeletal maturity. The clinical signs and symptoms may include limping, characterized by a shortened stance phase on the involved side; pain referable to the groin, trochanter region, or anterolateral thigh; guarding or spasm of the muscles around the hip joint; limitation of hip motion on passive examination; knee pain; and refusal to walk. Careful examination will often reveal atrophy of the thigh or buttock muscle, or both, as well. An extremely sensitive test is simply to have the patient lie supine on the examining table and, with the patient as relaxed as possible, gently to roll the involved limb from side to side. Involuntary muscle guarding, even of mild degree, is often readily detectable with this maneuver when compared with the response on the normal side.

Laboratory evaluation of patients with synovitis of the hip usually has negative findings but often must be done in order to help exclude acute infectious or metabolic processes. The complete blood count, sedimentation rate, and results of examination and culture of joint fluid are normal.

Radiographic examination will show no positive findings in most cases. Occasionally, one sees diminution of the definition of soft tissue planes around the hip joint or slight demineralization of the bone of the proximal femur, particularly in the metaphyseal region (Fig. 4–32).

Management of synovitis of the hip in-

Figure 4–32. Normal extracapsular fat lines. These may bulge or disappear with synovitis of the hip.

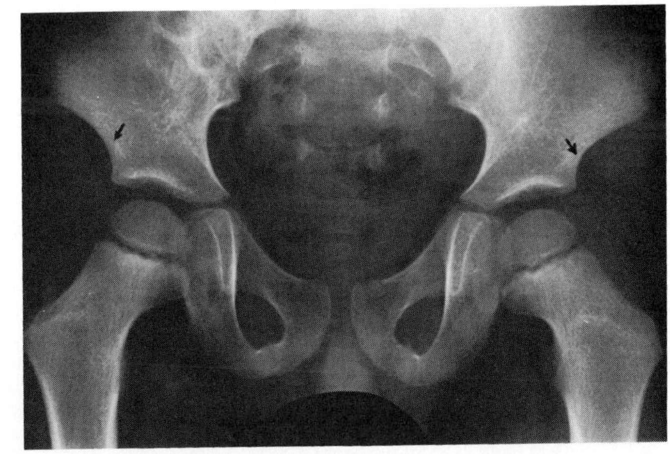

cludes, first and foremost, repeated examinations at intervals of a few days and often repeated radiographs or a bone scan in order to rule out a more serious pathologic process. This is critically important because the signs and symptoms of synovitis may be identical to those of infection, SCFE, Legg-Perthes disease, or neoplasia. The symptomatic patient is best treated with restriction of activities, ranging from use of crutches for walking to complete bed rest and traction if the pain and spasm are sufficiently severe.

The usual course of synovitis of the hip is gradual resolution of symptoms within two to three weeks. Analgesics are usually not necessary during the course of treatment. It cannot be emphasized too strongly that one must be certain to rule out more serious problems, which could have damaging effects on the hip joint.

References

Congenital Dysplasia of the Hip

Chunard EG and Logan ND: Varus-producing and derotational subtrochanteris osteotomy in the treatment of congenital dislocation of the hip. J Bone Joint Surg 45A:1399, 1963.

Coleman SS: Congenital Dysplasia and Dislocation of the Hip. St. Louis, CV Mosby Co, 1978.

Gage JR and Winter RB: Avascular necrosis of the capital femoral epiphysis as a complication of closed reduction of congenital dislocation of the hip. J Bone Joint Surg 54A:343, 1972.

Hensinger RN: Congenital dislocation of the hip. Ciba Found Symp Vol 31, No 1, 1979.

Howorth B: Development of present knowledge of congenital displacement of the hip. Clin Orthop 125:68, 1977.

Leveuf J: Primary congenital subluxation of the hip. J Bone Joint Surg 29:149, 1947.

Ozonoff MB: Controlled arthrography of the hip: A technique of fluoroscopic monitoring and recording. Clin Orthop 93:260, 1973.

Putti V: Congenital dislocation of the hip. Surg Gynecol Obstet 42:449, 1926.

Renshaw TS: Inadequate reduction of congenital dislocation of the hip. J Bone Joint Surg 63A:1114, 1981.

Salter RB and Dubos JP: The first 15 years personal experience with innominate osteotomy in the treatment of congenital dislocation of the hip. Clin Orthop 98:72, 1974.

Von Rosen S: Diagnosis and treatment of congenital dislocation of the hip joint in the newborn. J Bone Joint Surg 44B:284, 1962.

Wilkinson JA: Prime factors in the etiology of congenital dislocation of the hip. J Bone Joint Surg 45B:268, 1963.

Coxa Vara

Amstutz HC and Wilson PD Jr: Dysgenesis of the proximal femur (coxa vara) and its surgical management. J Bone Joint Surg 44A:1, 1962.

Blockey NJ: Observation on infantile coxa vara. J Bone Joint Surg 51B:106, 1969.

Pylkkanen P: Coxa vara infantum. Acta Orthop Scand [Suppl] 48, 1960.

Schmidt TL and Kalamchi A: The fate of the capital femoral physis and acetabular development in developmental coxa vara. J Pediatr Orthop 2:534, 1982.

Weinstein JN et al.: Congenital coxa vara: A retrospective review. J Pediatr Orthop 4:70, 1984.

Proximal Femoral Focal Deficiency

Aiken GT: Proximal Femoral Focal Deficiency: A Congenital Anomaly. Washington, National Academy of Sciences, 1969.

Fixsen JA and Lloyd-Roberts GC: The natural history of early treatment of proximal femoral dysplasia. J Bone Joint Surg 56B:86, 1974.

Koman LA et al.: Proximal femoral focal deficiency: A 50-year experience. Dev Med Child Neurol 24:344, 1982.

Panting AL and Williams PF: Proximal focal femoral deficiency. J Bone Joint Surg 60B:46, 1978.

Pappas AM: Congenital abnormalities of the femur and related lower extremity malformations: Classification and treatment. J Pediatr Orthop 3:45, 1983.

Septic Arthritis and Osteomyelitis

Fabry G and Meire E: Septic arthritis of the hip in children: Poor results after late and inadequate treatment. J Pediatr Orthop 3:461, 1983.

Griffin PP and Green WT: Hip joint infections in infants and children. Orthop Clin North Am 9:123, 1974.

Morrey BF et al.: Suppurative arthritis of the hip in children. J Bone Joint Surg 58A:388, 1976.

Nade S: Choice of antibiotic management of acute osteomyelitis and acute septic arthritis in children. Arch Dis Child 52:679, 1977.

Obletz BE: Acute suppurative arthritis of the hip in the neonatal period. J Bone Joint Surg 42A:23, 1960.

Tetzloff TR et al.: Oral antibiotic therapy for skeletal infections of children. II. Therapy of osteomyelitis and suppurative arthritis. J Pediatr 92:485, 1978.

Trueta J: Three types of acute hematogenous osteomyelitis. J Bone Joint Surg 41B:671, 1959.

Legg-Perthes Disease

Catterall A: Legg-Calve-Perthes Disease. Edinburgh, Churchill Livingstone, 1982.

Cotler JM: Surgery in Legg-Calve-Perthes syndrome. American Academy of Orthopaedic Surgeons Instructional Course Lectures 25:135, 1976.

Katz JF: Late modelling changes in Legg-Calve-Perthes disease with continuing growth to maturity. Clin Orthop 150:115, 1980.

Lloyd-Roberts GC et al.: A controlled study of the indications for and the results of femoral osteotomy in Perthes disease. J Bone Joint Surg 58B:31, 1976.

Salter RB: The present status of surgical treatment for Legg-Perthes disease. J Bone Joint Surg 66A:961, 1984.

Salter RB and Thompson GH: Legg-Calve-Perthes disease. The prognostic significance of the subchondral fracture and a two group classification of the femoral head involvement. J Bone Joint Surg 66A:479, 1984.

Weinstein SL: Legg-Calve-Perthes Disease. American Academy of Orthopaedic Surgeons Instructional Course Lectures 32:272, 1983.

Wynne-Davies R: Some etiologic factors in Perthes disease. Clin Orthop 150:12, 1980.

Slipped Capital Femoral Epiphysis

Aadalen RJ et al.: Acute slipped capital femoral epiphysis. J Bone Joint Surg 56A:1473, 1974.

Boyer DV et al.: Slipped femoral capital epiphysis: Longterm follow-up study of one hundred twenty one patients. J Bone Joint Surg 63A:85, 1981.

Gage JR et al.: Complications after cuneiform osteotomy for moderately or severely slipped capital femoral epiphysis. J Bone Joint Surg 60A:157, 1978.

Howorth B: History: Slipping of the capital femoral epiphysis. Clin Orthop 48:11, 1966.

Howorth B: Treatment: Slipping of the capital femoral epiphysis. Clin Orthop 48:53, 1966.

Jacobs B: Diagnosis and natural history of slipped capital femoral epiphysis. American Academy of Orthopaedic Surgeons Instructional Course Lectures 21:167, 1972.

Kramer WG et al.: Compensating osteotomy at the base of the femoral neck for slipped capital femoral epiphysis. J Bone Joint Surg 58A:796, 1976.

Melby A et al.: Treatment of chronic slipped capital femoral epiphysis by bone-graft epiphyseodesis. J Bone Joint Surg 62A:119, 1980.

O'Brien ET and Fahey JJ: Remodeling of the femoral neck after in-situ pinning for slipped capital femoral epiphysis. J Bone Joint Surg 59A:62, 1977.

Rao JR et al.: The treatment of chronic slipped capital femoral epiphysis by biplane osteotomy. J Bone Joint Surg 66A:1169, 1984.

Wilson PD et al.: Slipped capital femoral epiphysis: An end result study. J Bone Joint Surg 47A:1128, 1965.

Synovitis

Adams JA: Transient synovitis of the hip joint in children. J Bone Joint Surg 45B:471, 1963.

deValderrama JAF: The "observation hip" syndrome and its late sequelae. J Bone Joint Surg 45B:462, 1963.

Hardinge K: The etiology of transient synovitis of the hip in childhood. J Bone Joint Surg 52B:100, 1970.

Nachemson A and Scheller S: A clinical and radiographic follow-up study of transient synovitis of the hip. Acta Orthop Scand 40:479, 1969.

Neuhauser EBD and Wittenborg MH: Synovitis of the hips in infancy and childhood. Radiol Clin North Am 1:13, 1963.

Spock A: Transient synovitis of the hip joint in children. Pediatrics 24:1042, 1959.

5

The Lower Extremity and the Knee

In children's lower limbs, congenital anomalies and developmental variations are seen more commonly than are traumatic lesions. Many of these problems are obvious and easily recognizable, while others are subtle or may represent normal variations.

CONGENITAL PROBLEMS OF THE KNEE AND LEG

Congenital Dislocation or Hyperextension of the Knee

This is a rare anomaly. It is more common in females and is almost always bilateral. It may be associated with oligohydramnios, fibrosis of the quadriceps muscle, or congenital absence of the cruciate ligaments, or with such syndromes as sacral agenesis or arthrogryposis multiplex congenita. At least half the patients will have other musculoskeletal problems, the most common being dislocation of the hip. There is a spectrum of clinical appearances ranging from mild hyperextension of the knee to severe hyperextension with complete anterior dislocation of the tibia from the distal femur (Fig. 5–1). Excluding those children with neurologic disease, the cause is thought to be related to frank breech intrauterine positioning.

After searching for other anomalies or problems, the physician should begin treatment on the day of birth or as soon thereafter as possible. When treatment is started early, results are surprisingly good, and residual deformity or interference with function is unusual. Early treatment consists of passive stretching exercises, followed by gentle flexion to bring the knee into as much flexion as possible. The achieved correction is held with light plaster casts or splints. Manipulation should be carried out daily until bilateral flexion of more than 90 degrees can be achieved. Then it is wise to continue treatment with use of a Pavlik harness for a period of at least two months. If treatment is delayed, or if the child is not seen until later in infancy, then longitudinal skin traction for several days or weeks will be necessary as a preliminary means of realigning the tibia on the femur before flexion is started. If adaptive changes, such as soft tissue contractures in the anterior knee and fibrosis of the quadriceps muscle, have occurred, surgical release will be necessary.

Congenital Dislocation of the Patella

Because the neonatal patella is not ossified and is often difficult to palpate through the usual amount of prepatellar fat, this condition is not often diagnosed in the neonatal period. The clinical presentation is inability to extend the knee actively against gravity. Passive extension is possible, however, to the

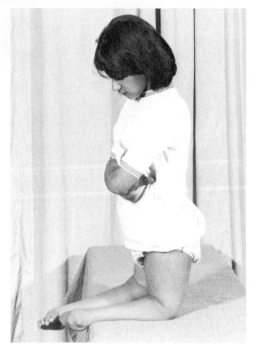

Figure 5–1. Severely neglected, bilateral congenital genu recurvatum with associated clubfoot deformities.

deformities being the most common. Other common findings are tarsal coalition, opposite foot deformities, and dysplasia of the hip. The condition is a longitudinal deficiency with either an intercalary or a terminal deficit. Severe involvement is more common than is mild. The clinical presentation is mild to marked shortening of the involved leg, often with flexion contracture of the knee. The foot may be normal or may be fixed in mild to severe varus. Absence of one or more rays is common.

Treatment depends upon the severity of the condition. In the severest cases with little or no proximal tibia and no functional quadriceps, knee disarticulation with subsequent prosthetic fitting is the treatment of choice. In patients with a normal distal femur, fair quadriceps function, but a very hypoplastic proximal tibial anlage and mild flexion contracture, a procedure to centralize the fibula can be considered. Some cases will later require amputation of the foot and orthotic control of the knee. In milder cases, the proximal tibia is essentially normal, and quadriceps function is also normal. Knee flexion contractures respond to serial casting, and the foot may be treated appropriately.

limit of the normal neonatal knee flexion contracture, which may be up to 20 degrees. Patellar dislocation may be associated with Down's syndrome, congenital dislocation of the knee, and other syndromes in which multiple dislocations occur.

Treatment of this condition by means of closed reduction and then immobilization is uniformly unsuccessful, since the patella and quadriceps slip off the femoral trochlea as soon as the reduction manipulation is released. Surgical treatment is necessary if the child will have the potential to walk. This consists of proximal realignment of the patella with lateral release and medial soft tissue advancement of the vastus medialis to the patellar periosteum. Quadriceps lengthening may also be necessary.

Congenital Absence or Deficiency of the Tibia (Tibial Hemimelia)

The severity of this condition ranges from hypoplasia of the distal tibia to total absence of the tibia with severe foot deformities (Fig. 5–2). About 20% of the cases are bilateral. Tibial hemimelia is associated with a high incidence of other anomalies, upper limb

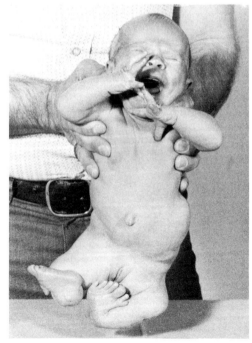

Figure 5–2. Bilateral absence of the tibia. There are severe varus deformities of both feet and ankles, and polydactyly on the left foot.

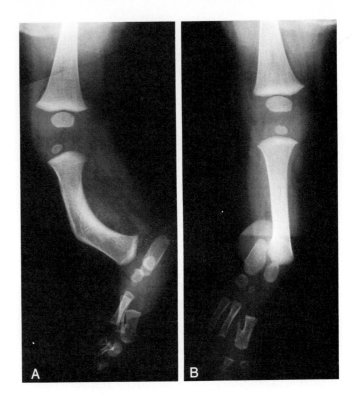

Figure 5–3. *A* and *B*, Congenital absence of the fibula. Note anterior bowing of the tibia and absence of the lateral rays of the foot.

Congenital Absence or Deficiency of the Fibula (Fibular Hemimelia)

This is more common than tibial hemimelia and is a longitudinal deficiency that may be either intercalary or terminal. It is the most common congenital limb deficiency. Many variations are possible. The fibula may be partially or totally absent, and this condition may be associated with multiple other limb problems, including bowing or shortening or both, of the tibia and defects of the femur (Fig. 5–3). Proximal focal femoral deficiency occurs in 10% to 20% of patients with fibular hemimelia.

The condition is slightly more common in males and is most often unilateral. The clinical presentation is shortening of the involved leg with bowing of the tibia and slight shortening of the femur, although more profound femoral deficit may be present. The foot deformity is often severe and consists of equinus, valgus, and absence or abnormality of the lateral rays. A skin dimple is common at the apex of the tibial bowing. In many cases, there is a palpable tight fibrous band running from the posterolateral proximal tibia to the heel, which represents the fibular anlage.

Treatment of fibular hemimelia is ex-tremely complex and must be individualized. Most of the severe forms will require foot amputation in order to give the patient a stable platform on which to walk and to correct the limb length inequality.

Congenital Posteromedial Bowing of the Tibia

This condition is noted at birth and is characterized by shortening and bowing of the tibia in a convex posteromedial direction, with the posterior component predominating (Fig. 5–4). The foot is in a calcaneovalgus position. Bilaterality is rare.

The treatment of posteromedial bowing is manipulation and casting to correct the deformed foot. This is almost always successful. Rarely is specific treatment necessary for the tibial bowing, since this corrects spontaneously with growth and most cases are fully straight by the time that the patient is two or three years old. Orthoses are unnecessary, and osteotomy is extremely rarely indicated. The ultimate significance of this condition is the leg length inequality. The eventual discrepancy is predictable early in life, since it continues as a constant percentage of the normal limb. Epiphyseodesis to retard the

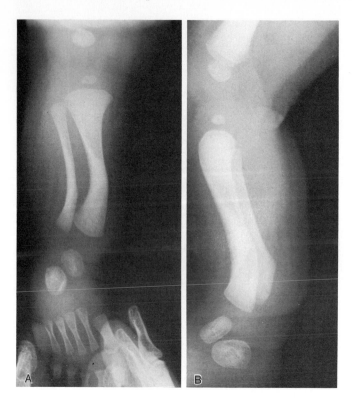

Figure 5–4. *A,* Posterior medial bowing of the tibia as seen on the AP view. *B,* Lateral view demonstrating the posterior bowing.

growth of the longer leg is necessary if the predicted discrepancy exceeds two centimeters. This can be properly timed by consulting the appropriate growth charts. Only infrequently does the discrepancy reach four or five centimeters. If it does, tibial lengthening should be considered.

Congenital Anterior Bowing and Congenital Pseudarthrosis of the Tibia

Anterior bowing is far different from posteromedial bowing. It carries a different prognosis, and depending on the severity, it is usually a much more difficult problem.

In very mild cases, there is slight anterior bowing of both the tibia and the fibula. The fibula is otherwise normal. There may also be mild shortening of the tibia. These cases should be followed carefully. While the majority will correct spontaneously, some will stabilize, and some will become progressively deformed. Those that stabilize can be safely treated with realignment osteotomy done at an older age.

Those that bow progressively have a poor prognosis (Fig. 5–5). Cyst formation and ob-

literation of the medullary canal of the bone are the rule, with increasing bowing and ultimately pathologic fracture occurring early in childhood. It is wise to protect these with an orthosis prophylactically to attempt to prevent fracturing. When a fracture occurs, it is very difficult to treat. Nonunion is a common occurrence. With modern techniques of internal fixation, bone grafting, and electrical stimulation, the outlook is now much better than it had been in the past. These cases will still require lifelong orthotic protection.

The most severe variant of anterior bowing is congenital pseudarthrosis of the tibia, with marked anterolateral bowing being obvious at birth. More than 50% of patients with this anomaly have neurofibromatosis (Fig. 5–6). At birth, either a fracture is already present (10% to 20%) or there is a profound narrowing at the junction of the proximal two thirds and the distal third. The fibula is also abnormal at this level. Although 75% of those that fracture do so by the time that the patient is two years old, the fracture may occur at any time during life. Once union has been obtained, it is difficult to maintain, even with orthotic protection. Although continuous protection with an orthosis may seem some-

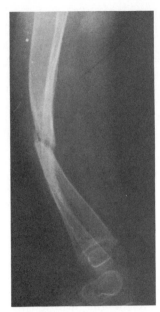

Figure 5–5. Congenital pseudarthrosis of the tibia. Note the anterior bowing and the abnormal bone quality in the tibial shaft.

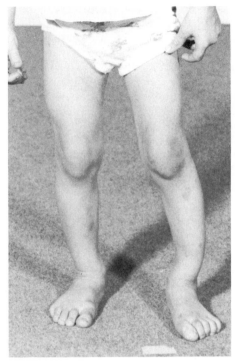

Figure 5–6. Congenital pseudarthrosis of the left tibia in a patient with neurofibromatosis.

what drastic, it is preferable to multiple surgical attempts at obtaining union. In the most severe cases, or when a reasonable attempt at obtaining union has failed, it is in the child's best interest to consider strongly conversion to a below-knee amputation and fitting of a prosthesis.

Congenital Annular Bands

This condition is discussed in Chapter 2. Annular bands in the lower extremity may be unilateral or bilateral (Fig. 5–7). They

may occur anywhere in the limb but are more common distally and are often associated with a clubfoot and with edema distal to the band. Treatment is described in Chapter 2.

INTOEING

Intoeing is the most common orthopedic reason for a child to present at a medical

Figure 5–7. Congenital annular bands (Streeter's dysplasia) involving the right lower extremity. The left toes are also involved.

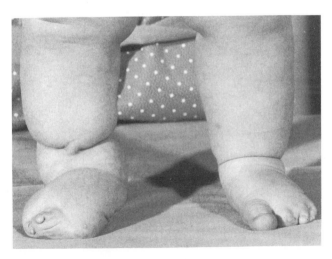

practitioner's office accompanied by concerned parents or grandparents or both. It is essential to determine the cause of intoeing. This is easily accomplished by clinical examination alone.

The major causes of intoeing are femoral anteversion, internal tibial torsion, and problems of the foot. The latter include clubfoot, medial deviation of the talar neck, metatarsus varus, overactive abductor hallucis, and dynamic intoeing. Conditions occurring in the foot are discussed in Chapter 6.

Excessive Femoral Anteversion

Femoral anteversion is a normal anatomic condition in which the femoral neck is angled forward or anteriorly from the femoral shaft in response to forces around the hip and lower extremity. Anteversion allows a maximum amount of hip rotation while preserving stability in flexion, which is necessary for sitting. With excessive femoral anteversion, when the child stands the lower extremity rotates internally to seat better the femoral head into the acetabulum, and intoeing occurs.

The normal amount of femoral anteversion is approximately 50 degrees at birth, and it decreases by about two degrees per year to reach a normal range of 15 to 20 degrees at skeletal maturity. The underlying cause of excessive femoral anteversion is increased ligamentous laxity, whereby the anterior capsule of the hip joint fails to provide a stable buttress against the anteverted femoral head. This buttressed pressure is necessary for the normal gradual remodeling of anteversion to occur. With the overly lax capsule of the hip, increased anteversion is allowed to persist. This results in the so-called "anteversion syndrome," characterized by ligamentous laxity and significant intoeing with internal rotation of the entire lower extremity. Also part of the syndrome are flexible flat feet, caused by both the laxity and the body's corrective tendency to pronate the foot in order to compensate for intoeing; genu recurvatum or "back-knee," which is secondary to laxity; and an increase in lumbar lordosis as the pelvis tilts forward in an attempt to cover the femoral head (Fig. 5–8). A later compensatory mechanism for femoral anteversion is the development of more-than-normal external tibial torsion.

A pathognomonic sign of anteversion is abnormal rotation of the hips, which should be examined in extension (Fig. 5–9). Normally, in younger children external rotation exceeds internal rotation, and then at maturity the ranges are approximately equal. With excessive anteversion, internal rotation markedly exceeds external rotation. The abnormal range includes up to 90 degrees of internal rotation and 30 degrees or less of external rotation.

A potential problem with anteversion, in addition to the cosmetic effect on gait, is that in severe cases patellofemoral rotational malalignment can occur with patellofemoral instability and early degeneration of the patellofemoral joint. There is also a theoretical possibility that maldistributed forces across the hip joint are generated, and early degenerative arthritis of the hip may occur. The patient who is likely to have problems in adult life is the one whose anteversion is greater than 50 degrees (measured on radiographs) and who has 80 degrees or more of internal rotation and less than 15 degrees of external rotation of the hip in extension. In reality, very few patients have anteversion of this severe a magnitude.

Because of the rarity of severe anteversion and because of the tendency for anteversion of less severe magnitude (less than 50 to 60 degrees) to remodel or be compensated for during growth, parental reassurance is all that is necessary for the vast majority (greater than 99%) of the patients with excessive anteversion. Attempts at correction of anteversion with the use of corrective footwear, twister cables, or other types of orthoses have universally failed. The only effective treatment is surgical correction by employment of derotation osteotomies of the femora.

Corrective osteotomy is indicated in children older than the age of five years when spontaneous remodeling or compensation has failed to occur and when severe anteversion persists. These four findings should all be present: 80 degrees or greater of internal hip rotation; less than 10 to 15 degrees of external rotation; severe cosmetic gait deformity; and the absence of compensatory external tibial torsion. The corrective surgery involves performance of a supracondylar osteotomy of the distal femur with cross-pin internal fixation and then immobilization in a spica cast six weeks. After the age of 9 or 10 years, compensatory external tibial torsion is usually advanced, and derotation osteotomy may be contraindicated. It bears reem-

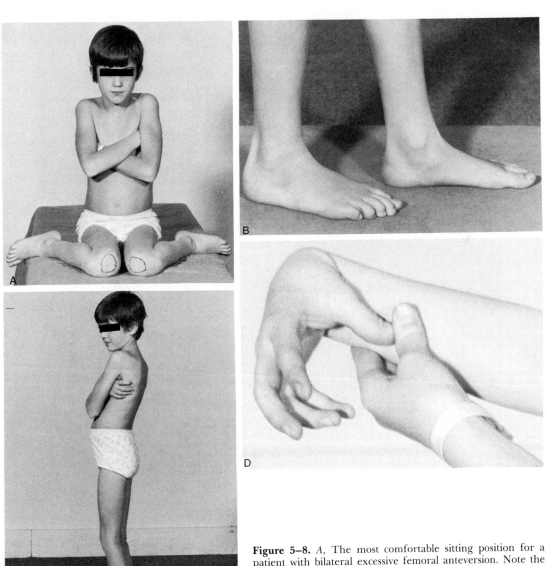

Figure 5–8. *A,* The most comfortable sitting position for a patient with bilateral excessive femoral anteversion. Note the extreme internal rotation of the femora. *B,* This girl has bilateral planovalgus feet, which are almost always seen in association with femoral anteversion. *C,* Lumbar hyperlordosis with femoral anteversion is secondary to anterior tilting of the pelvis in an effort to cover the femoral head. *D,* Ligamentous laxity is the rule in patients with excessive femoral anteversion.

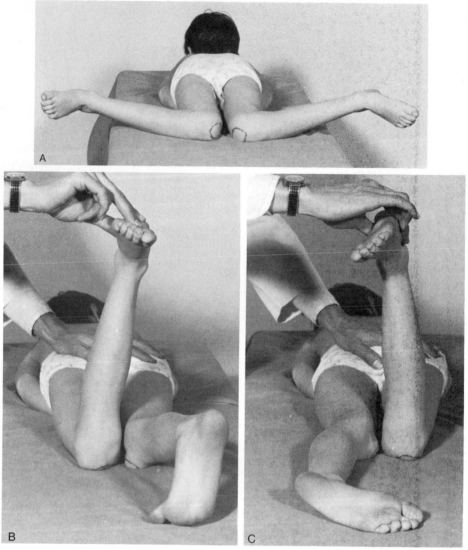

Figure 5–9. *A*, Examination with the hips in extension shows almost 90 degrees of internal rotation bilaterally. *B*, Maximum external rotation on the left is zero degrees. *C*, Maximum external rotation on the right is zero degrees.

phasizing that less than one per cent of all patients with femoral anteversion are seriously considered for surgical treatment.

Internal Tibial Torsion

Children are normally born with internal tibial torsion of 0 to 20 degrees. This is determined by measuring the axis of ankle motion and the bimalleolar axis of the ankle against the axis of knee flexion and extension. Although there are complex and expensive radiographic means of measurement that are more precise, clinical estimation is per-

fectly adequate. The natural history of internal tibial torsion is slow derotation with growth, particularly during the first seven years. The normal range of adult external tibial torsion is 0 to 40 degrees, with an average of approximately 20 degrees. Although significant internal tibial torsion produces an intoeing type of gait, it is extremely rare to see tripping or mild sprains and strains of the ankle secondary to this condition.

More than 99% of children with internal tibial torsion will experience satisfactory correction as a result of growth alone. Before the age of two years, correction can probably be accelerated by the use of night splints. Splinting can range from simply tying the heels of a pair of shoes together to using a Denis Browne bar. Alternatively, one can attempt to prevent the child from spending excessive amounts of time sitting on the lower extremities with the legs internally rotated. Probably fewer than one case per thousand will need derotation osteotomy of the distal tibia because of the persistence of severe internal tibial torsion into late childhood. Shoe modifications have no effect on tibial torsion at any age.

OUTTOEING

As with intoeing it is important to find the cause of outtoeing. There are three common ones: (1) External rotation contracture of the hip in infancy; (2) femoral retroversion, seen in early childhood; and (3) external tibial torsion, seen in later childhood (much less common).

External Rotation Contracture of the Hip

External rotation contracture of the hip is a common neonatal finding. It is secondary to persistent tightness in the external rotator muscles due to intrauterine positioning. In this condition, both lower extremities are externally rotated, with the knees pointing outward. Examination of the hips in extension with the patient lying prone shows very little internal rotation and marked external rotation, sometimes in excess of 90 degrees. This condition usually persists through the first 12 to 18 months of life, being corrected by the stretching out of the external rotator muscles by reciprocal crawling and later by reciprocal walking. Surgical correction of this condition has not been necessary in the 88-year existence of the Newington Children's Hospital.

Femoral Retroversion

Femoral retroversion is the opposite of excessive femoral anteversion and is extremely rare. Whereas external rotation contracture of the hip is detected during infancy and has usually disappeared completely by walking age, femoral retroversion is rarely noted until the child has gained proficiency

in independent ambulation. The child presents with external rotation of the entire lower extremity during walking, with the patellae facing outward. Retroversion is confirmed by noting the abnormal hip rotation in extension, with external rotation usually exceeding internal rotation by a factor of three or more. Management of this condition includes documenting the degree of retroversion with radiographic examination and then allowing the mechanisms of growth to remodel the disorder or compensate for it. A busy pediatric orthopedic surgeon will probably complete his entire professional career without having to perform derotation osteotomy for this condition.

External Tibial Torsion

External tibial torsion is much less common than internal torsion and is exceedingly rare in pure form (Fig. 5–10). It is most often a compensatory mechanism for excessive femoral anteversion. When polio was prevalent, it was common to see external tibial torsion secondary to contractures to the iliotibial

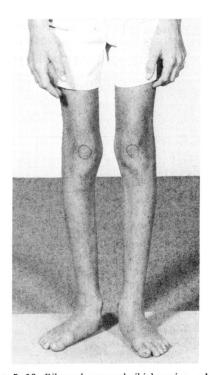

Figure 5–10. Bilateral external tibial torsion, which is more pronounced on the right. Note that both knees are pointing straight ahead.

band and of the tensor fascia lata musculature. Isolated external tibial torsion is almost
never severe enough to require surgical correction. If detected early, night splinting and
avoidance of prolonged sitting with the tibiae
externally rotated may be beneficial.

KNOCK-KNEES AND BOWLEGS

Knock-knee (genu valgus) and bowleg
(genu varus) are part of the pattern of normal lower limb development. Most children
are born with mild to moderate varus (15
degrees), but by the age of 18 to 24 months
the legs are essentially straight. Then, by the
age of three, overcompensation into valgus
of an average of about 12 degrees has occurred. With further growth, the normal five
to eight degrees of valgus seen in adults is
reached, usually by the age of seven years.

Genu Valgus or Knock-knee

Genu valgus is classified as apparent, physiologic, or pathologic. The latter two types
are usually accompanied by mild external
tibial torsion. Apparent knock-knee may be
due to fat thighs, increased joint laxity, or
hypotonia. When the angle between the thigh
and the leg is measured, it falls within the
normal range for the patient's age.

Physiologic or idiopathic genu valgus represents the overwhelming majority of cases
of knock-knee seen in physicians' offices. Approximately 20% of all three-year-olds have
more than 15 degrees of valgus; however,
only one per cent of these will have a persis-
tently high degree of valgus after the age of
seven years (Fig. 5–11).

The best approach to the child with knock-
knees is to obtain radiographs the lower extremities with the patient in a standing position to rule out disease of the knee joint and
to allow accurate measurement of the angle.
It is important that the film be taken with
the knees and the feet pointing straight
ahead, since rotation can markedly alter the
measured angle. Spontaneous improvement
with further growth can then be documented. Occasionally, physiologic genu valgus becomes significant enough to produce a
cosmetic deformity or unequal stress across
the two sides of the knee joint or both. The
potential exists for early degenerative arthritis to develop on the lateral side of the knee.
This occurs in less than one per cent of

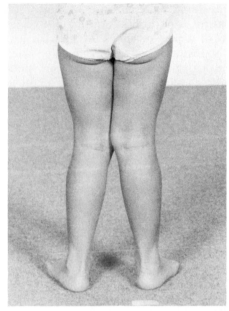

Figure 5–11. Bilateral genu valgus of moderate degree
in a three-year-old girl. This condition corrected spontaneously.

children, so it is important to remember that
physiologic knock-knee resolves spontaneously. Therefore, for almost all patients,
any form of treatment is both ineffective and
unnecessary. A time-honored myth is that a
medial heel wedge on the shoe will correct
knock-knee by transmitting more force to the
medial side of the knee and slowing growth
This is physiologically and biomechanically
impossible and is a waste of money. For the
rare exception—an older child who has
greater than eight centimeters' distance between the medial malleoli at the ankles when
standing with knees together—one should
consider distal medial femoral epiphyseodesis or stapling to allow retardation of medial growth, persistence of lateral growth,
and spontaneous correction. This is usually
done by about the age of 10 or 11 years in
girls, and 12 to 13 years in boys.

Pathologic genu valgus may be caused by
paralytic conditions, juvenile rheumatoid arthritis, rickets, trauma, endocrine abnormalities, infections in the proximal tibia or distal
femur, and Hubner's disease, which is a rare
tibial cause of genu valgus. Any of these
conditions can produce a valgus knee, which
rarely improves with growth and may require
osteotomy, growth plate stapling, or epiphyseodesis.

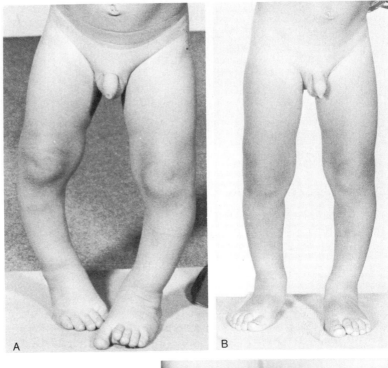

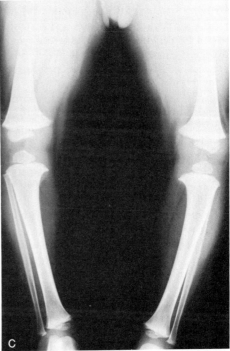

Figure 5–12. *A*, Bilateral physiologic genu varus. *B*, Fifteen months later, marked spontaneous improvement has occurred. *C*, Bilateral physiologic genu varus. Note the beaking of the metaphysis of the distal femora and proximal tibiae. This condition subsequently resolved spontaneously.

Genu Varus or Bowleg

Most genu varus seen by health practitioners is physiologic and corrects spontaneously (Fig. 5–12). It is detected shortly after birth and may persist up to two years as a normal variant. Bowlegs may also be caused by a pathologic entity known as "Blount's disease" or by other pathologic processes. Any type of genu varus is usually accompanied by internal tibial torsion.

Physiologic bowleg is normal at birth. In

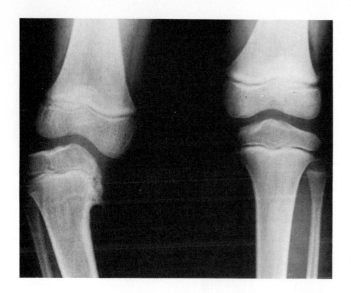

Figure 5–13. Blount's disease involving the right proximal tibia.

cases with 15 degrees or less of bowing, all that is needed is serial documentation of improvement. If greater than 15 degrees is present, then one should consider a Denis Browne bar, used during naps and at night, with the feet set much greater than shoulder width apart and the bar bent into a caudally directed convexity. This will allow more rapid correction by increasing the pressure on the lateral side of the knee to retard lateral growth, via the Heuter-Volkmann principle, at the lateral proximal tibial and distal femoral physes. Children younger than the age of two years will usually tolerate this type of treatment. After age two, when the child possesses the fine motor coordination needed to remove the bar and use it as a boomerang, it will fail.

Some cases of physiologic bowing are progressive. These are usually associated with the following conditions: early walking, infantile obesity, increased internal tibial torsion, and an overly wide-based gait as a toddler. Consistently increased force on the medial side of the knee is the result, with subsequent injury to the epiphysis, the growth plate, and the metaphysis, and progressive varus deformity in the proximal tibia (Fig. 5–13). This is known as Blount's disease or tibia vara.

Blount's Disease

Blount's disease occurs most commonly between the ages of one and four years and is bilateral in about half the cases. It is slightly more common in females. When progressive genu varus is noted, treatment should be instituted. If the child is younger than the age of two years, bracing with a Denis Browne bar or a knee-ankle-foot orthosis may be effective. If progression continues or if the child is older than the age of two, however, then proximal tibial osteotomy is indicated. If surgery is delayed, permanent growth plate damage may occur, which may necessitate repeated osteotomies or more extensive surgery such as growth plate resection with inert spacer interpositioning to attempt to prevent recurrence. It is far better to intervene before permanent damage has occurred.

A second type of Blount's disease occurs in obese juveniles or adolescents whose legs have been previously in slight varus. It probably represents a similar disease process. This is much less common than infantile tibia vara, is usually milder (less than 20 degrees), and is most often unilateral and accompanied by mild shortening of the tibia. Many cases regress spontaneously. Proven progressive cases are best treated by performance of an osteotomy.

LOWER LIMB LENGTH INEQUALITY (ANISOMELIA)

Although no one is exactly bilaterally symmetric, and all of us have some minor variation in the lengths of our limbs, nevertheless there are several conditions that can produce significant limb length inequality in the lower extremities. The problem with significant limb length inequality, defined as greater than two centimeters in an average-sized adult, is that if uncorrected, it can lead to an unsightly limp, increased energy consumption during walking, scoliosis in the lower spine, and occasional low back pain. Limb length discrepancy in the arms is a different matter. It is rarely of any functional significance, and only if severe is it a cosmetic problem. The major impact of upper extremity limb-length inequality is that one has an ongoing need for the services of a good tailor or seamstress.

In managing lower limb length inequality, it is important to document serially the precise lengths of the lower limbs. Clinical assessment of lower limb length discrepancy is best done by measuring the extended lower limb from the anterior superior iliac spine to the tip of the medial malleolus. If the foot is deformed, then the distal limit should be the plantar surface of the os calcis. There are several radiographic ways of documenting inequality, the best probably being the scanogram, in which the hip joint, knee joint, and ankle joint are seen on a single film that contains a metric scale. The resultant discrepancy can be plotted on a temporal graph. Then tables of height, limb length, predicated growth, and ultimate discrepancy are consulted, the best-known being those of Green and Anderson and of Moseley. All data are based upon skeletal age, not chronologic age. Skeletal age is determined by comparing the radiographic appearance of the wrist (assuming that the wrist is normal) with the illustration in the standard atlas developed by Greulich and Pyle.

Congenital Hemihypertrophy

In this condition, the extremities on one side of the body are increased in length and circumference. Conditions such as neurofibromatosis, hemangiomas, arteriovenous fistulas, and other vascular problems should be ruled out. In idiopathic hemihypertrophy, the percentage of discrepancy usually remains constant during growth, which is helpful in predicting the ultimate discrepancy and planning any needed correction.

Associated problems have been reported with hemihypertrophy. These include neo-plasms in the liver, kidney, and adrenal glands and renal anomalies such as polycystic kidneys and Wilms' tumor. Three per cent of Wilms' tumors occur in patients with hemihypertrophy. Therefore, when this condition is identified, a renal work-up is in order.

Congenital Hemiatrophy

This condition is sometimes difficult to differentiate from hemihypertrophy (Fig. 5–14). If one limb appears to be disproportionately large or disproportionately small, the diagnosis is easy. Hemiatrophy most likely represents an idiopathic hypoplasia of one limb with decreased length and girth. Other anomalies are rarely found associated with it. These patients need similar follow-up and planning to that required for those with hemihypertrophy.

Neurofibromatosis

Neurofibromatosis, or Von Recklinghausen's disease, is frequently associated with

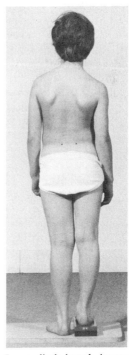

Figure 5–14. Lower limb length inequality caused by idiopathic right-lower extremity hemiatrophy. Note the presence of compensatory scoliosis despite leveling the pelvis with wooden blocks. Equalization of lower limb lengths was achieved by means of epiphyseodesis of the left distal femur and proximal tibia.

enlargement of one limb. Any organ in the body may be involved. An in-depth discussion of neurofibromatosis is beyond the scope of this text. It is important to note, however, that with limb length discrepancy in neurofibromatosis, growth patterns are often unpredictable.

Silver's Syndrome

Infants with Silver's syndrome are smaller at birth and shorter than normal as adults. Anisomelia caused by hemihypertrophy is a constant finding. Most patients have a retarded skeletal age, and, in some, increased gonadotropin levels have been found in the urine. Scoliosis may develop, and, less commonly, syndactyly is also seen. Treatment of limb length discrepancy by standard methods is successful in Silver's syndrome.

Trauma

Fractures of the femur in children between the ages of two and nine years frequently result in overgrowth of the involved limb, the average amount being about one centimeter. Because of this, most orthopedic surgeons elect to reduce these fractures with 1 centimeter of overriding (bayonet) apposition. Fractures of the tibia do not often cause overgrowth, but if they do, the overgrowth is of lesser magnitude.

Depending upon the anatomic pattern of the fracture, injuries to growth plates, can produce growth arrest owing to direct irreparable damage to the cells of the growth plate itself or to cross-union of the epiphysis to the metaphysis. Obviously, the younger the child when growth plate arrest occurs, the greater the discrepancy. Not only linear but also angular discrepancy should be expected and appropriately treated. Any time a fracture involves a physis, the child's parents should be counseled about possible future growth disturbance.

Klippel-Trenaunay Syndrome

This syndrome consists of multiple vascular anomalies, including arteriovenous fistulas, cutaneous hemangiomas, varicose veins, and marked hypertrophy of all tissues in the involved limb or part of a limb. It is unilateral

in 90% of cases. Profound overgrowth can occur in this condition and may be accompanied by high-output cardiac failure. Treatment is exceptionally difficult, and the majority of patients are best managed by modifying their footwear. In mild cases, the careful use of elastic stockings or leotards is of benefit. In more severe instances, epiphyseodesis or even amputation may be considered.

Infection

The infection that has resulted in more anisomelia than any other is poliomyelitis. Many polio patients were left with some degree of limb length inequality. The treatment of asymmetry after poliomyelitis is often complicated by the associated muscle weakness, which may be profound and often requires use of an orthosis to counter the motor loss and to control joint instability. When orthotics are needed, a shoe lift is an excellent means of equalizing limb lengths.

Other infectious processes, such as septic arthritis or osteomyelitis, can produce limb shortening through direct damage to epiphyses or growth plates. Neonatal staphylococcal sepsis has a particular penchant for destroying the hip and also the distal femoral physis. Conversely, limb overgrowth may happen when metaphyseal osteomyelitis and concomitant increased vascularity are present a significant period of time.

Hip Problems

Lower limb length discrepancies may result from avascular necrosis in a child's hip, either associated with congenital hip dysplasia or owing to Legg-Perthes disease. Coxa vara is another cause of anisomelia. Conditions such as slipped capital femoral epiphysis or fractures around the hip rarely cause significant inequality, unless avascular necrosis ensues.

Treatment of Limb Length Inequality

The options for treatment of anisomelia include: accepting the discrepancy, which is appropriate if the ultimate difference is two centimeters or less; lengthening the short side; or shortening the long side. The simplest means of "lengthening" the short side

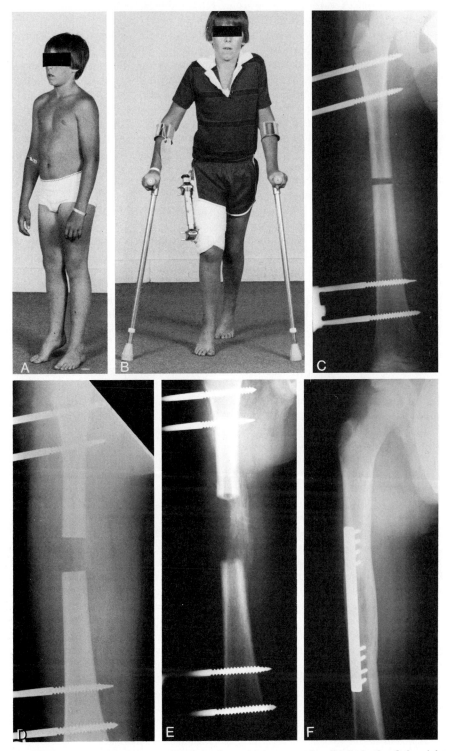

Figure 5–15. *A,* Marked limb length inequality secondary to trauma to the distal physis of the right femur. The patient was treated with right femoral lengthening. *B,* During the lengthening procedure, the patient was able to walk with crutches. Note the lengthening device lateral to the right thigh. *C* to *F,* Sequential radiographs of the procedure for lengthening the right femur. Gradual distraction is accomplished by means of an external fixator at the rate of 1 to 1.5 mm of distraction per day. Following completion of the distraction, some early healing is noted. At that point, the external fixator is replaced with a plate, and the gap is reinforced with autogenous bone graft.

is to build up the shoe. A one-half to one centimeter lift can be placed inside the heel of most shoes without interfering with the shoe's fit or function, but more lengthening than this requires augmentation of the heel and sole. More than two centimeters of augmentation may be unsightly. In adolescents and adults, the compliance with shoe augmentation varies inversely with the amount of lift applied.

Lengthening the shorter side is accomplished by means of division of the bone at the midshaft, metaphysis, or growth plate and slow distraction to a desired length, often followed by internal fixation and bone grafting (Fig. 5–15). This is a reasonable and effective method but entails a substantial amount of careful orthopedic surgical management. It is most successful when the limb is otherwise normal. Prerequisites for lengthening include a strong bone, absence of fixed joint contractures, absence of infection, absence of neurovascular compromise, and normal joints at each end of the bone to be lengthened. As a rule of thumb, 20% to 25% of the original length of the bone can be gained at each lengthening.

Shortening of the involved limb is most easily accomplished during the growth period by simply destroying a growth plate. This is known as epiphyseodesis. Charts and tables for predicting the amount of growth remaining, based on bone age, are available, and precise calculations can be made. This is an excellent means of limb length equalization and is the most commonly used form of treatment. If the patient's growth has been completed, then shortening of the longer side can be accomplished by excising a segment from an area of the bone where union is expected to be rapid and then applying internal fixation. This is also a precise and effective way of equalization.

Other methods, such as attempting to stimulate the growth of the bone through the production of vascular shunts or fistulas or through local inflammatory reactions, have been very unsuccessful and are contraindicated. Current research on the use of electrical currents or pulsating electromagnetic fields to stimulate growth is inconclusive at present. For anisomelia that is severe and that involves significant anomalies and deformities of the shortened limb, amputation and fitting of a prosthesis is often the best solution.

KNEE PROBLEMS

Pain in the knee area is a common complaint in children. Although the patellofemoral joint, the tibiofemoral joint, or the surrounding soft tissues are most often the source of the disorder, it is critical to remember that major hip disease such as tumors, slipped epiphyses, and Legg-Perthes disease frequently presents as pain in the region of the knee. Tunnel vision, therefore, can be disastrous.

Patellofemoral Problems

The patella is a sesamoid bone whose main mechanical function is to increase the lever arm of the quadriceps or knee extensor muscle group. It also functions to centralize the pull of the quadriceps; to resist friction and compression of the quadriceps tendon as it passes over the knee joint; to protect the anterior knee as a bony shield; to bear weight during kneeling or knee-walking; and, finally, at least in some people's judgment, to be a positive cosmetic factor. The posterior surface of the patella contains the thickest articular cartilage in the body and covers the subchondral bone, in which pain fibers run. It is interesting to note that when one is walking with the knee flexed at 10 degrees, approximately half the body weight is transmitted to the patellofemoral joint. When climbing stairs with the knee flexed at 60 degrees, a force of three and one-third times body weight is exerted on the patellofemoral joint, and during deep knee bends more than seven times body weight can be transmitted to the retropatellar surface.

The major patellofemoral problems seen in children are related to malalignment and instability (Fig. 5–16). Symptoms of malalignment and instability of the patellofemoral joint include pain, particularly when climbing stairs or during knee bends; intermittent giving way or buckling of the knee; crepitation at the patellofemoral joint; occasional swelling; and a feeling of stiffness or "catching" in the knee. True locking of the knee (inability to extend fully) is rare with patellofemoral disease and is more often a sign of a meniscus disorder.

Patellofemoral pain is probably caused by either increased intraosseous pressure or subchondral bone microfractures. The latter re-

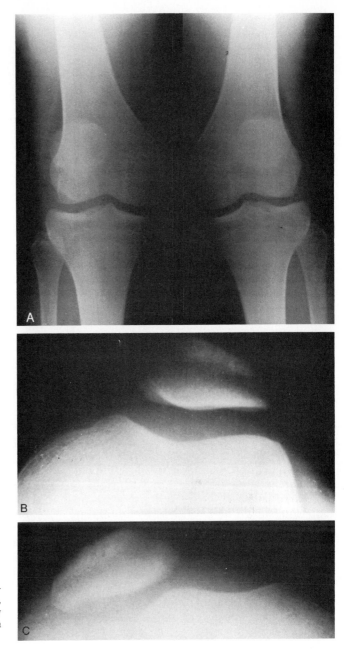

Figure 5–16. *A,* AP view of both knees showing lateralization of both patellae. *B* and *C,* Tangential views in 30 degrees of flexion show the right patella to be stable *(B),* the left patella dislocated *(C).*

sult from increased pressure on one side of the patella, usually the lateral side, due to lateral tracking of the patella (malalignment) during flexion and extension of the knee. Such lateral tracking may be the result of medial soft tissue laxity; a high-riding patella or patella alta secondary to tightness of the rectus femoris muscle; tightness of the tensor fascia lata or iliotibial band, or both, which produces a lateral tethering effect; increased valgus at the knee, or femoral anteversion,

which can increase the lateral quadriceps vector.

Positive diagnostic signs include atrophy of the vastus medialis part of the quadriceps; tightness of the rectus femoris or the iliotibial band, or both; patella alta; increased genu valgus; femoral anteversion; pain on palpation of the retropatellar facets; and crepitation on compression of the patella against the femoral trochlea. Chondromalacia is characterized by softening, fissuring, fibrillation, and fragmentation of the retropatellar articular cartilage. It results from chronic excessive pressure. Tangential axial ("sunrise") radiographs of the patellofemoral joint with the knee in various degrees of flexion are often helpful. Both knees should be viewed simultaneously so that comparisons can be made.

Increased lateral pressure responds best to a program of exercises designed both to stretch the tight rectus and iliotibial band and to strengthen the quadriceps muscle, particularly the vastus medialis part, and the medial hamstrings. If no degenerative changes are present, then isotonic exercises, through a full range of knee motion, are the treatment of choice. With significant degenerative changes and pain, isometric exercises with the knee at or near full extension are probably more appropriate. If exercises fail, a lateral soft-tissue release may be considered.

Patellar Subluxation or Dislocation

Patellofemoral subluxation or dislocation or both, can be the result of isolated instances of trauma or simply severe malalignment over a long period of time. This condition occurs most commonly between the ages of 10 and 25 years, with a peak at age 15. It is three times more common in girls. Patients with subluxation usually show the signs of increased lateral pressure and also a positive Fairbank sign. This is elicited by attempting to displace the patella laterally. A positive result is a marked increase in the patient's apprehension, often to the point where she will grab the examiner's hand. Patellofemoral subluxation often responds to an exercise program, the principles of stretching and strengthening being the same as in the treatment of lateral pressure. If an adequate exercise program is not successful, surgical realignment procedures are appropriate.

Patellofemoral dislocation due to acute trauma carries an unfavorable prognosis, and without adequate treatment in the initial episode, at least 85% of cases will recur. The first acute dislocation should be treated by splinting the knee in extension at least three to four weeks, followed by an aggressive muscle rehabilitation program. Chronic recurrent subluxation or dislocation requires surgical treatment by either proximal realignment or distal realignment (or both).

Plica

A plica is an abnormal membranous, curtainlike structure that originates in the suprapatellar synovial recess and extends downward, usually on the medial side of the knee joint. It can become entrapped between the femur and the tibia. This results in pain, a sensation of giving way, and occasionally locking of the knee. It is easily diagnosed with arthrography or arthroscopy. When recurrent symptoms are a problem, arthroscopic excision of the plica affords relief.

Fat Pad Syndrome or Hoffa's Disease

This condition is characterized by pain in the anterior knee, just posterior to the patellar ligament between the inferior patella and the tibial tubercle. The pain is intermittent and is sometimes accompanied by mild swelling. The retropatellar fat pad becomes enlarged and tender and may even be compressed or pinched in between the tibia and the femur. Treatment consists of rest, splinting, or relief from weight bearing until symptoms subside. Partial excision of the fat pad is very rarely necessary.

Discoid Lateral Meniscus

This is a congenital anomaly that usually produces no symptoms in early childhood, although it may cause a clicking or snapping sensation on the lateral side of the knee (Fig. 5–17). Later, pain and swelling and occasional locking of the knee may occur, and lateral joint-line tenderness is common. The diagnosis is confirmed by means of arthrography or arthroscopy. Whether the lesion should be partially or totally excised depends on the magnitude of the disease. Total lateral meniscectomy in a child may result in early degenerative arthritis of the lateral side of the knee.

Internal Derangement

Internal derangement most often refers either to a torn meniscus or cruciate ligament or to a loose body in the knee joint. Meniscal tears are usually the result of trauma and

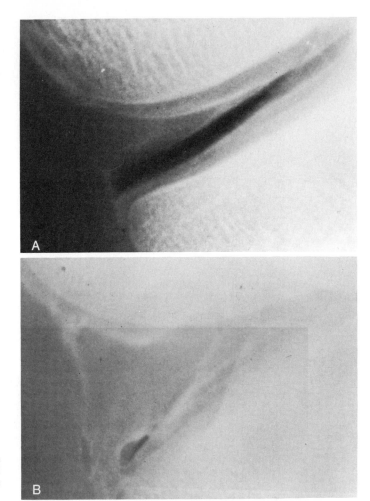

Figure 5–17. *A,* Arthrographic view of a normal medial meniscus. *B,* A discoid lateral meniscus of the same knee. Note the increased thickness and irregularity.

present with a history of locking, giving way, pain, and intermittent swelling. No longer is a torn meniscus an indication for total meniscectomy. With advances in arthroscopic surgery, partial meniscectomy and, in some cases, peripheral meniscal repair should produce better long-term results and should decrease the incidence of osteoarthritis of the knee.

A loose body in the knee joint may be the result of a small articular surface fracture, but often no history of trauma can be elicited. Synovial chondromatosis produces multiple loose bodies. A loose body in the knee joint produces intermittent symptoms of instability, pain, and swelling and locking of the knee—similar if not identical to those of meniscal disease. When loose bodies are identified, they should be removed to prevent damage to the articular surfaces.

Osteochondritis Dissecans

This is an osteocartilaginous lesion, most commonly occurring on the medial femoral condyle (Fig. 5–18). It is probably caused by single or repeated trauma to the partially flexed knee, which results in a compression fracture due to impingement by the tibial spine. Alternatively, it may be produced by compression from the medial side of the patella. Osteochondritis dissecans is more common in boys. The condition is occasionally bilateral. Often the lesion is asymptomatic, but it may present with poorly localized knee pain, occasional mild effusion, and even symptoms of giving way or locking. In most cases, the cartilaginous articular surface is intact, although partial or complete detachment of the osteochondral fragment may occur. A free fragment in the knee joint

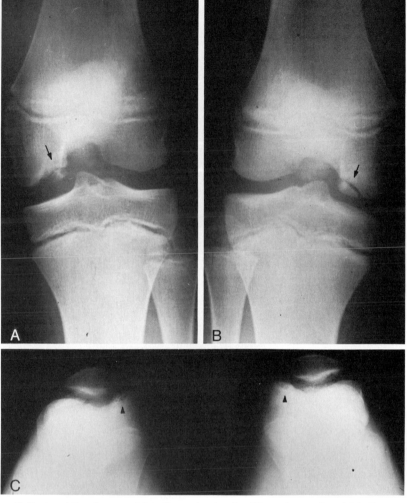

Figure 5–18. *A to C,* Flexion AP and tangential radiographs showing bilateral osteochondritis dissecans of the medial femoral condyles.

produces symptoms of repeated locking, giving way, pain, and effusion.

The treatment for lesions in continuity consists of restricting activities to the patient's tolerance level. Healing can be expected over a period of several months. If healing does not occur, a period of immobilization of the knee is appropriate. If there is any question about the fragment being a loose body in the knee, arthroscopic examination is appropriate. Small loose fragments should be removed from the knee joint, whereas large fragments with significant bony components should be replaced in their osseous bed and secured with internal fixation. Osteochondritis dissecans is extremely rare in adults.

Osgood-Schlatter Disease

Osgood-Schlatter disease is a condition of traumatic overuse of the tibial tubercle, caused by repeated microtrauma. Either there is a microtearing of the fibers of insertion of the quadriceps tendon from the bony epiphysis, of which the tubercle is a part, or else the lesion is a partial separation through the growth plate. In either event, the result is a painful enlargement of the tubercle. The pain is increased by strenuous physical activity. This condition occurs during preadolescence and adolescence and is more common in males.

Radiographic studies are not usually nec-

ing function of the knee joint, but more commonly it is due to the bowstring snapping of a tendon over a condylar bony prominence. The most common is snapping of the popliteus tendon over the lateral femoral condyle. A less common cause of snapping knee is ligamentous laxity, which allows rotary subluxation of the tibia on the femur.

The asymptomatic snapping knee is best managed by reassurance, although further investigation is necessary if symptoms of pain or swelling are present or develop. A discoid lateral meniscus may require surgical treatment. If the popliteus tendon is found to be the cause, however, then tenotomy (although not often needed) is curative and produces no functional loss. Ligamentous laxity may improve with growth and maturity, but a knee orthosis may be required in the interim.

Popliteal Cyst (Baker's Cyst)

This lesion is a cystic mass filled with clear thick fluid. It occurs most often in boys. The cyst arises either as an isolated sac from the semimembranosus bursa or as a herniation of the synovial membrane between the semimembranosus tendon and the origin of the medial head of the gastrocnemius muscle. Although it may become quite large, it rarely causes pain or other symptoms (Fig. 5–20).

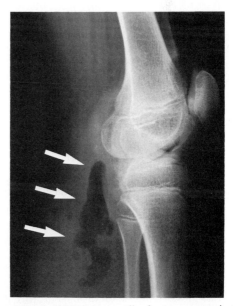

Figure 5–20. This large popliteal cyst communicated with the knee joint and partially filled with air during arthrography.

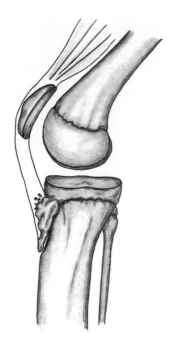

Figure 5–19. Osgood-Schlatter disease. The tibial tubercle is irregular and fragmented.

essary and may show completely negative findings in the early stages. Later, there may be evidence of slight avulsion or fragmentation of the tubercle, or both (Fig. 5–19). In some cases, ossicles form in the quadriceps tendon just above its attachment.

This condition is most often a very benign one and is often completely asymptomatic. In those patients who have persistent or recurrent pain, restriction of activities to tolerance levels and the occasional use of mild analgesics are appropriate. In more severe cases, immobilization of the knee with relief from weight-bearing, if needed, is effective. Osgood-Schlatter disease may be episodic with recurrences throughout adolescence, but nearly all cases cease to be symptomatic at the time of the closure of the proximal tibial growth plate. On rare occasions, painful bony fragments persist in the tendon and require surgical excision.

Snapping Knee

Children sometimes present with a snapping sensation in the region of the knee joint that does not cause pain but is often quite disconcerting to the parents. The phenomenon may be caused by a discoid lateral meniscus, which interferes with the smooth glid-

A popliteal cyst in a child is usually a self-limited condition, and the majority will resolve spontaneously and will completely disappear over a period of a few months to a few years. Attempts at surgical excision are usually unnecessary and may result in recurrence. In adults, this lesion is associated with an extremely high incidence of intra-articular disease, but this is not the case in children, and further investigation of the knees of asymptomatic children with popliteal cysts is probably not warranted. Transillumination of the cyst is usually all that is required to confirm the diagnosis. Needle aspiration in an attempt to cure this lesion has proved futile.

INFECTIONS AROUND THE KNEE

Osteomyelitis

Osteomyelitis in the lower extremity occurs most commonly around the knee. There is often an association between recent trauma to the knee region and the development of bone infection. Eighty-five per cent of all osteomyelitis occurs in patients younger than 16 years of age, with a male-to-female ratio of four to one. The portal of entry is usually the blood stream, except in cases of contaminated open wounds or local extension from a nearby infected focus. The most common cause of osteomyelitis at any age, but particularly after the age of two years, is *Staphylococcus aureus*.

The vascular anatomy of bone is a major determinant of the clinical presentation and pathologic severity of osteomyelitis. During the first 12 to 18 months of life, the growth plates are traversed by vascular channels of communication between epiphysis and metaphysis. This offers little resistance to the extension of an infection of the distal end of a bone. After the age of 18 months and until its closure, the growth plate acts as a barrier, the vascular channels having dropped out, and most infections are localized to either the metaphyseal or, much less commonly, the epiphyseal region (Fig. 5–21). When skeletal maturity is reached, vascular continuity between the epiphysis and metaphysis is reestablished.

Once a contained metaphyseal infection erodes through the thin bony cortex, whether septic arthritis ensues is dependent upon whether the metaphysis is intra- or extracap-

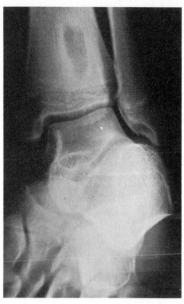

Figure 5–21. Osteomyelitis of the distal tibial metaphysis. This produced slight overgrowth but early physis closure.

sular. The distal femoral and proximal tibial metaphyseal regions are extracapsular. The infection is shunted across the thin metaphyseal cortex, erodes the bone in that region, and extends into the subperiosteal space. Since children have a very thick but very loosely applied periosteum, the untreated infection dissects in the subperiosteal space and is contained. Therefore, large areas of involvement with new periosteal bone formation (involucrum) are seen. When the original central bone is infarcted, the affected area is called the sequestrum. Although the knee joint is not infected, a sterile effusion is common.

The presenting clinical signs of osteomyelitis include malaise, fever, anorexia, muscle spasm or guarding around the knee, localized tenderness, and pseudoparalysis (unwillingness to move the leg). Localized edema and erythema may also be present. Local calor is usually detectable. Laboratory studies show increase in the erythrocyte sedimentation rate (ESR), anemia, and a normal or increased white blood count with a shift to the left. Other sources of infection should be sought, blood cultures should be done, and appropriate orifices should also be cultured. It is frequently appropriate to perform needle aspiration of the metaphysis, the direct approach to bacteriologic diagnosis. A bone scan will help in ruling out other areas of involvement or metastatic lesions.

The radiographic diagnosis depends upon the stage of the pathologic process. The first sign is loss of soft tissue planes, usually occurring within three to five days. Between 7 and 12 days, some mottling of the bone density is seen. Next, periosteal changes with new bone formation occur peripherally, with central bony destruction continuing. Finally, chronic osteomyelitis is established, characterized by sequestrum and involucrum formation.

The treatment of acute osteomyelitis is based upon identification of the causative organism. Immediate intravenous administration of appropriate antibiotics in adequate dosage should be begun. Administration of antibiotics should be continued until the ESR has returned to normal. A common regimen is five days of intravenous treatment, after which oral administration should begin. With oral administration of antibiotics, the bacteriocidal serum levels should be monitored. In the acute phase, bed rest, immobilization, analgesics, and hydration are also important and, if needed, surgical decompression. Surgical decompression is performed in acute osteomyelitis to drain suspected pus under pressure in order to prevent further necrosis or to obtain a diagnosis when other attempts have failed. Decompression is accomplished by making a small incision in the skin and then a small window in the periosteum and cortical bone. Then curettage of material for culture and irrigation of the wound are performed. Healing is by secondary intent. Chronic osteomyelitis, on the other hand, is treated only by surgical means. It requires excision of devitalized tissue and sequestra, provision of adequate drainage, and either primary closure over suction–irrigation tubes or healing by secondary intent. In more severe cases, muscle-pedicle or free-vascularized muscle flaps may be very helpful.

Septic Arthritis

Septic arthritis is a true emergency (Fig. 5–22). Approximately two thirds of all cases occur before the age of three years, and it is more common in males. Eighty per cent of the cases involve joints of the lower extremity. The mechanism of onset is usually hematogenous dissemination of organisms to the synovial membrane and thus into the knee joint itself. Direct extension of osteomyelitis through the growth plate via vascular channels, through the epiphysis, and into the joint may occur before the age of 18 months. The clinical presentation is a warm, painful, tender joint with muscle spasm and pseudoparalysis. The infant may show no early signs other than irritability and poor feeding.

Laboratory findings include a marked increase in the ESR, usually with a normal white blood count, but anemia is often present. The diagnosis is confirmed by (1) aspirating purulent fluid from the joint and obtaining positive results of a joint fluid smear or culture, (2) discovering a high white blood cell count in the joint fluid (100,000 per cubic milliliter or greater), and (3) seeing blood cultures with positive findings. The early radiographic changes are capsular distention and, occasionally, widening of the joint space. As the process continues, joint destruction and narrowing may be seen.

The treatment of septic arthritis of the knee consists of adequate surgical drainage and appropriate intravenous antibiotic therapy. Early splinting is necessary for comfort, but motion should be reinstituted as rapidly as possible in order to improve the functional

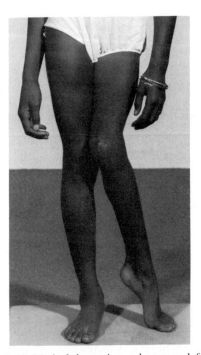

Figure 5–22. Marked shortening and rotatory deformity secondary to septic arthritis of the left knee. Damage to the joint and the distal femoral and proximal tibial physis is present.

result. Although some physicians advocate simple repeated aspirations as an adequate means of draining the joint, one is always impressed at the time of arthrotomy at the amount of necrotic material, fibrin clot, and other debris that can be easily washed from the joint by means of a simple, straightforward arthrotomy. Temporarily leaving a small drain in place assures decompression of the joint and egress of the infectious process on a continuing basis. The direct injection of antibiotics into septic joints is not only unnecessary but is contraindicated.

LEG PAINS

Leg pains are common in children and may result from any of a broad spectrum of causes. These range from highly malignant bone tumors to occasional mild discomfort of unknown cause that disappears spontaneously. The differential diagnosis includes neoplasia, trauma, collagen diseases, vascular problems, metabolic disorders, infections, muscle compartment syndromes, and psychogenic factors. The proper approach to the child with leg pains is a thorough history, a physical examination, radiographic studies, and laboratory studies, if indicated. The three most common causes of leg pain in children are growing pains, shin splints, and stress fractures.

Growing Pains

Growing pains occur in approximately 10% of the pediatric population and are slightly more common in females. They tend to occur in "pain prone" families. Probably 90% to 95% of all leg pain in children falls into this category. "Growing pains" is actually a misnomer, since the onset is usually after the age of three years, not during the period of most rapid growth. In fact, growth probably plays no role whatsoever in the development of this condition. Nevertheless, the term is well entrenched and need not be dislodged from the medical lexicon. It is rare for the discomfort to persist beyond the age of 12 years.

Growing pains are characterized by intermittent aching in the muscles of the leg or the thigh, usually described as being deep in the limb and not near the joints. They may last a few minutes to several hours and occur most commonly in the late evening or after bedtime, but they disappear by morning. The pains are often severe enough to wake the child from sleep and are more common in cold or wet weather. They are also more common in children with emotional disturbances. During the day, the child demonstrates no limp or decreased activity. The pains are usually bilateral. It is not unusual to see abdominal pain or headaches, or both, associated with the leg pain. There is no history of significant trauma. The result of a physical examination is entirely negative, as are laboratory and radiographic findings. In fact, the cause is usually unknown, although myriad hypotheses are available. In some cases, pronated feet or tight heel cords, or both, are associated with growing pains. Treatment of foot disorders may therefore resolve the problem.

Treatment of growing pains is highly empirical and usually consists of massage, application of heat (such as wearing two pairs of pajama pants to bed), use of mild analgesics such as acetaminophen, reassurance that there is no serious organic cause, and periodic reevaluation at intervals of 6 to 12 months to assure that an early pathologic lesion has not been missed. In intractable cases, evaluation for family disturbances by a competent psychologist is sometimes very rewarding.

Shin Splints

Shin splints are characterized by substantial pain along the medial or lateral tibial shaft. Symptoms are usually most prominent after running or other physical activity, especially in the spring and summer after a winter of relative inactivity. The cause is overuse with repetitive stress leading to such things as microtears in muscle, tendon, or ligament groups; muscle inflammation; inflammation at the tendon-bone junction; periostitis; and mild muscle compartment syndromes. In muscle compartment syndromes, repetitive trauma produces edema in the muscle compartment with increased pressure and a cycle of venous and arterial occlusion, increased ischemia, increased occlusion, and, in severe cases, both muscle and nerve fiber necrosis. Mild cases of compartment syndromes respond to rest. In moderate to extreme cases, a surgical emergency exists requiring decompression of all involved compartments.

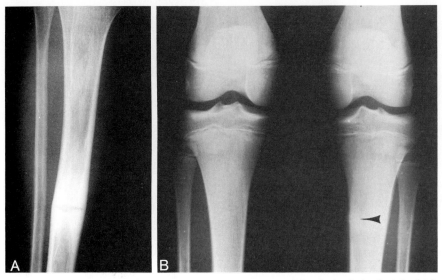

Figure 5–23. *A,* Stress fracture of the right tibial shaft. *B,* This boy complained of pain in the left tibial region. Note the stress fracture, as indicated by the arrow.

The treatment for milder types of shin splints begins with rest until the patient is asymptomatic. Then a graduated program of progressive exercise and activity is instituted. The use of ice and mild analgesics may also be helpful. Other modalities of physical therapy are probably unnecessary. There are definite situations in which poor footwear and running on improper surfaces are also factors in the development of shin splints.

Stress Fractures

Stress fractures may be insidious and yet may cause severe leg pain. They are most common in the tibia and can occur anywhere throughout the length of the bone, including the metaphyseal region, although diaphyseal stress fractures are more common (Fig. 5–23). They may also occur in the fibula and in the femur. Stress fractures present with pain that increases with increasing activity and is localized to the site of the lesion. Ordinary radiographic views usually show negative findings until there is evidence of bone resorption and new bone formation, usually two weeks or longer following the onset of symptoms. A technetium bone scan shows positive results much earlier.

The treatment is rest, with or without immobilization. Most cases require at least three months of restricted activity and radiographic documentation of healing before ac-

tivity can be gradually resumed. A walking cast can often afford considerable relief.

TRAUMA INVOLVING THE FEMUR AND THE TIBIA

The Hip

Fractures and dislocations of the hip and fractures of the proximal femur are not common in children. Forces of substantial magnitude are required to produce them. Traumatic dislocation of the hip is very rare in children and usually is the result of an automobile accident (Fig. 5–24). With dislocation, the limb is shortened, adducted, and internally rotated, with flexion at the hip and the knee. Evaluation should include a careful search for other injuries in the trunk and the extremities, especially vascular and neurologic injuries in the lower limb. The next step is thorough radiographic evaluation, including computerized tomography, to assure that the injury is a pure dislocation and is not associated with fracture. Most pure dislocations can be treated with prompt closed reduction, whereas if fracture fragments are present, open reduction is usually necessary. The major complication from a dislocated hip is avascular necrosis of the femoral head, which is caused by disruption of the blood supply at the time of the injury. It may be unavoidable, although there appears to be a relationship between the length of time that

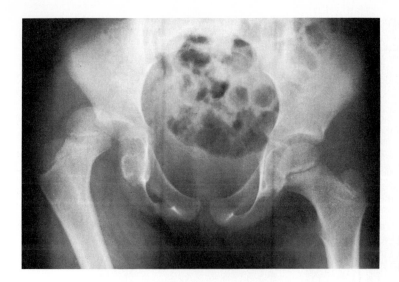

Figure 5–24. Traumatic dislocation of the right hip in a nine-year-old girl.

the dislocation persists before reduction and the development of avascular necrosis. Following prompt reduction, immobilization and relief from weight-bearing are necessary until soft tissue healing occurs.

Fractures in the proximal femur may occur through the growth plate, the femoral neck, or the intertrochanteric or subtrochanteric areas (Fig. 5–25). On clinical examination, these also show flexion, shortening, and pseu-

doparalysis with muscle spasm, but unlike dislocations, the limb is in external rotation. The risk of avascular necrosis is greater with fractures than with dislocation; in general, the more proximal the fracture in the proximal femur, the more likely the development of avascular necrosis. Treatment may consist of traction and immobilization in a cast for the intertrochanteric and subtrochanteric fractures. The majority of proximal femoral fractures, and virtually all femoral neck fractures, cannot be adequately managed by closed means and are best treated with open reduction, internal fixation, and often immobilization in a spica cast until healing occurs.

Fractures of the Shaft of the Femur

Diaphyseal fractures are common in children. Although they are frequently unstable, treatment is relatively simple because of the strong periosteal sleeve that can be used to help guide the fracture fragments into the desired position. The fracture is produced either by direct blunt trauma or by torsional forces, and an association with child abuse should always be considered (Fig. 5–26). The appearance of the fracture usually gives precise information regarding its cause. Direct blunt trauma produces transverse fractures, whereas oblique or spiral fractures are the result of twisting.

The treatment of femoral shaft fractures in children is nonoperative, usually beginning with appropriate traction to restore the desired length and alignment. It should be remembered that overgrowth of approxi-

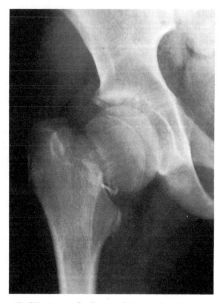

Figure 5–25. Acute fracture of the midneck of the right femur with posterior and inferior displacement. This injury requires open reduction and internal fixation, and the likelihood of avascular necrosis is substantial.

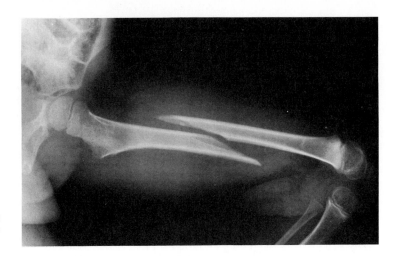

Figure 5–26. Spiral fracture of the diaphysis of the left femur secondary to child abuse.

mately one centimeter occurs in children between the ages of two and nine years. After two or three weeks of traction, there is usually sufficient early healing that reduction will not be lost if the patient is placed in a cast-brace or a hip spica cast and mobilized. Some fractures of the femur can be treated by means of immediate application of a cast-brace or spica cast, but this type of treatment requires very careful monitoring to assure that excessive shortening or recurrent angulation has not occurred. As with all major injuries, associated trauma to other systems should be suspected and ruled out. Of note is the fact that children and adults may lose 10% to 20% of their blood volume into the thigh from a single femoral fracture.

Fractures of the Distal Femur

Distal femoral fractures almost always involve the physis. A common fracture is a transverse separation through the growth plate that leaves a small triangular segment of the metaphysis attached to the distal fragment (Fig. 5–27). To minimize the risk of permanent growth plate injury, perfect reduction is essential. This is usually, but not always, possible by closed means. In spite of perfect reduction, the incidence of growth disturbance following fractures through the distal femoral physis in children is about 60%.

Dislocation of the Knee

Complete traumatic dislocation of the knee is exceedingly rare in children, being seen most often in adolescents whose growth plates have closed. This injury is often associated with severe neurovascular damage. Although salvage of the limb is possible, the amputation rate is high.

Dislocation of the Patella

This injury needs to be differentiated from the chronic unstable patellofemoral joint de-

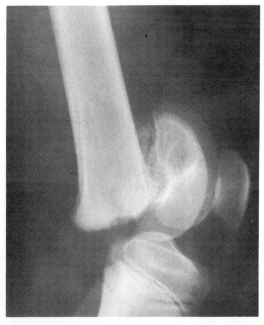

Figure 5–27. Fracture through the distal physis of the femur. There is a small attached metaphyseal fragment.

scribed previously. The treatment of acute dislocation consists of fully extending the knee, following which closed reduction is quite simple, and then immobilizing the knee at least three to four weeks to allow for soft tissue healing. In order to try to prevent recurrence, a program of muscle rehabilitation is essential, but even with such a program the recurrence rate is high.

Fractures of the Proximal Tibia

The proximal tibial growth plate has a tortuous, convoluted anatomy. It is very broad in surface area and has strong peripheral soft tissue attachments, including periosteum and ligaments. For these reasons, fracture through the proximal tibial growth plate is uncommon. When it does occur, it is usually the product of substantial force, so neurovascular injuries may be associated with it. The treatment is anatomic reduction, which may or may not be possible with closed manipulation, and adequate immobilization.

Avulsion of the tibial tubercle can occur as an isolated event, particularly after forceful flexion of the knee against a maximally contracted quadriceps muscle. This causes avulsion of not only the tibial tubercle but also the anterior portion of the epiphysis, of which the tubercle is a part. The displaced fragment requires operative replacement and internal fixation if it cannot be reduced by extension of the knee.

A special note should be made of valgus-angulated fracture of the proximal tibial metaphysis near its junction with the diaphysis (Fig. 5–28). This fracture most commonly occurs between the ages of two and eight years in males with pre-existing genu valgum. It is usually a transverse greenstick fracture of the medial cortex. In about 60% of cases, localized medial overgrowth into more valgus occurs. The excessive valgus will not be remodeled with growth and often requires an osteotomy for correction. Initial treatment of this seemingly innocuous fracture usually consists of, if possible, full or slight over-reduction, usually with the patient under

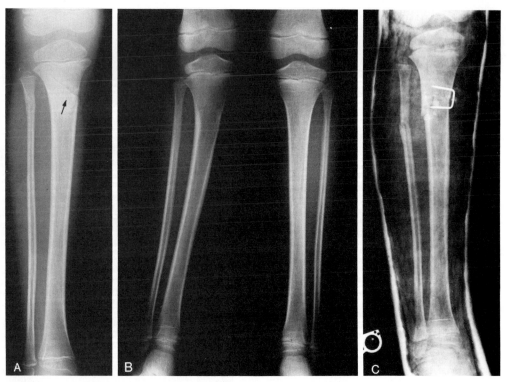

Figure 5–28. *A,* Incomplete fracture of the proximal medial right tibia. *B,* The result of the fracture was medial overgrowth and valgus angulation at the fracture site. *C,* A proximal tibial and fibular osteotomy was required to realign the leg.

general anesthesia, and use of a long-leg cast with the knee in extension. Six weeks are required for healing, during which time the reduction should be carefully monitored. The parents should be warned about the common occurrence of growth deformity after this fracture.

Tibial Shaft Fractures

The periosteal sleeve of a child's tibial shaft is exceptionally strong and usually prohibits the significant displacement of fractures in this region. Most are easily treated with

closed reduction and appropriate immobilization until healing has occurred. Open reduction of this fracture is almost never indicated in children.

Ankle Injuries

Isolated ankle dislocation is extremely rare in children, fractures being the rule because the ankle ligaments are stronger than the growth plates of the distal tibia and fibula. Diagnosis is not difficult, and precise radiographic documentation is easily obtainable.

Mild strains with minimal swelling or ten-

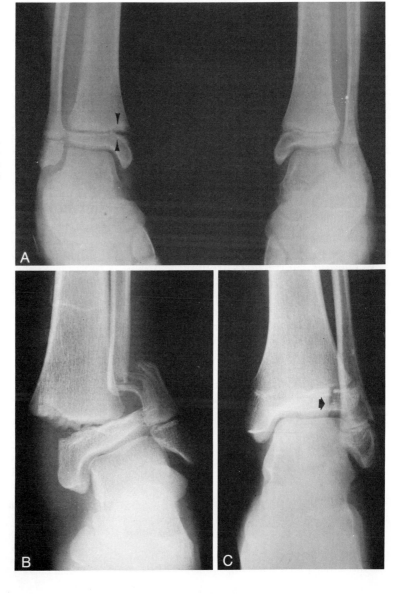

Figure 5–29. *A*, A nondisplaced fracture through the growth plate of the distal right tibia. Note slight widening of the plate. *B*, Fracture through the distal tibial growth plate and shaft of the distal fibula. The prognosis for continued growth of the distal tibia is uncertain, since crushing of the plate may have occurred. *C*, A fracture through the growth plate and epiphysis of the distal left tibia, with minimal displacement. This fracture is associated with a high incidence of premature closure of the physis.

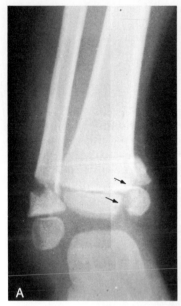 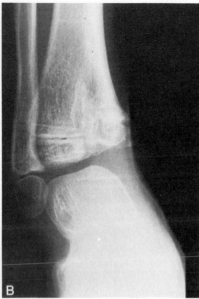

Figure 5–30. *A*, Fracture through the epiphysis, physis, and metaphysis of the distal right tibia with an associated transverse avulsion fracture through the distal fibula. *B*, This fracture resulted in premature partial closure of the distal tibial physis with progressive angular deformity. Complex reconstructive surgery was required.

derness respond to the use of soft compression dressings and crutches for 7 to 10 days. If there is greater swelling, a hematoma, and tenderness, but no fracture, it should be assumed that a ligament tear has occurred. Immobilization in a plaster cast is the safest and most comfortable means of treatment. This can be a walking cast, with weight-bearing allowed when the patient's discomfort permits. At least three weeks of immobilization will usually obviate chronic instability and the necessity for late reconstructive surgery.

In children, all fractures around the ankle involve one or more growth plates (Fig. 5–29). These require perfect anatomic reduction. While some types are amenable to simple closed treatment, others are very difficult to hold, and one should never hesitate to perform open reduction and internal fixation. Depending upon the age of the patient, adequate immobilization lasts four to six weeks. While healing is not a problem, the incidence of growth disturbance is high (Fig. 5–30).

References

Congenital Dislocation of the Knee and Patella

Curtis BH and Fisher RL: Congenital hyperextension with anterior subluxation of the knee. J Bone Joint Surg 51A:255, 1969.
Green JP and Waugh W: Congenital lateral dislocation of the patella. J Bone Joint Surg 50B:285, 1968.

Jones RDS et al.: Congenital dislocation of the patella. Clin Orthop 119:177, 1976.
Niebauer JJ and King DE: Congenital dislocation of the knee. J Bone Joint Surg 42A:207, 1960.
Nogi J and MacEwen GD: Congenital dislocation of the knee. J Pediatr Orthop 2:509, 1982.
Stem MB: Congenital dislocation of the knee. Clin Orthop 61:261, 1968.

Tibial Hemimelia

Brown FW: Construction of a knee joint in congenital total absence of the tibia (paraxial hemimelia, tibia). A preliminary report. J Bone Joint Surg 47A:695, 1965.
Jayakumar SS and Eilert RE: Fibular transfer for congenital absence of the tibia. Clin Orthop 139:97, 1979.
Jones D et al: Congenital aplasia and dysplasia of the tibia with intact fibula. Classification and management. J Bone Joint Surg 60B:31, 1978.
Wehbe MA et al: Tibial agenesis. J Pediatr Orthop 1:395, 1981.

Fibular Hemimelia

Farmer AW and Laurin CA: Congenital absence of the fibula. J Bone Joint Surg 42A:1, 1960.
Thompson TC et al.: Congenital absence of the fibula. J Bone Joint Surg 39A:1229, 1957.
Westin W et al.: Congenital longitudinal deficiency of the fibula. Follow-up of treatment of Syme amputation. J Bone Joint Surg 58A:492, 1976.

Congenital Posteromedial Bowing of the Tibia

Heyman CH et al.: Congenital posterior angulation of the tibia with talipes calcaneus. J Bone Joint Surg 41A:476, 1959.
Pappas AM: Congenital posteromedial bowing of the tibia and fibula. J Pediatr Orthop 4:525, 1984.

Congenital Pseudarthrosis of the Tibia

Masserman RL et al.: Congenital pseudarthrosis of the tibia. A review of the literature and 52 cases from the Mayo Clinic. Clin Orthop 99:140, 1974.

Nicoll EA: Infantile pseudarthrosis of the tibia. J Bone Joint Surg 51B:589, 1969.

Sofield HA: Congenital pseudarthrosis of the tibia. Clin Orthop 76:33, 1971.

Van Nes CP: Congenital pseudarthrosis of the leg. J Bone Joint Surg 48A:1467, 1966.

Femoral Anteversion

Fabry G et al.: Torsion of the femur—A follow-up study in normal and abnormal conditions. J Bone Joint Surg 55A:1726, 1973.

Somerville EW: Persistent foetal alignments. J Bone Joint Surg 39B:106, 1957.

Staheli LT: Torsional deformity. Pediatr Clin North Am 24:799, 1977.

Staheli LT et al.: Femoral anteversion and physical performance in adolescent and adult life. Clin Orthop 129:213, 1977.

Internal Tibial Torsion

Engel GM and Staheli LT: The natural history of torsion and other factors influencing gait in childhood. Clin Orthop 99:12, 1974.

Hutter CG Jr and Scott W: Tibial torsion. J Bone Joint Surg 31A:511, 1949.

Kling TF and Hensinger RN: Angular and torsional deformities of the lower limbs in children. Clin Orthop 176:136, 1983.

Ritter MA et al.: Tibial torsion. Clin Orthop 120:159, 1976.

Staheli LT and Engel GM: Tibial torsion: A method of assessment and a study of normal children. Clin Orthop 86:183, 1972.

External Rotation Contracture of the Hip

Pitkow RB: External rotation contracture of the extended hip. Clin Orthop 110:139, 1975.

Genu Valgus or Knock-Knee

McDade W: Bow legs and knock knees. Pediatr Clin North Am 24:825, 1977.

Salenius P and Vankka E: The development of the tibiofemoral angle in children. J Bone Joint Surg 57A:259, 1975.

Genu Varus or Bowleg or Blount's Disease

Blount WP: Tibia vara. J Bone Joint Surg 19:1, 1937.

Langenskiold A and Riska EB: Tibia vara (osteochondrosis deformans tibiae). J Bone Joint Surg 46A:1405, 1964.

O'Neill DA and MacEwen GD: Early roentgenographic evaluation of bowlegged children. J Pediatr Orthop 2:547, 1982.

Thompson GH et al.: Late onset tibia vara: A comparative analysis. J Pediatr Orthop 4:185, 1984.

Wenger DR et al.: The evolution and histopathology of adolescent tibia vara. J Pediatr Orthop 4:78, 1984.

Leg Length Inequality

Anderson M et al.: Growth and predictions of growth in the lower extremities. J Bone Joint Surg 45A:1, 1963.

Green WT and Anderson M: Epiphyseal arrest for the correction of discrepancies in the length of the lower extremities. J Bone Joint Surg 39A:853, 1957.

Greulich WW and Pyle SI: Radiographic Atlas of Skeletal Development of the Band and Wrist. Stanford, Stanford University Press, 1959.

Mathis TM and Bower JR: Tibial and femoral lengthening: A report of 54 cases. J Pediatr Orthop 2:487, 1982.

Moseley CF: A straight-line graph for leg length discrepancies. J Bone Joint Surg 59A:174, 1977.

Peterson HA: Partial growth plate arrest and its treatment. J Pediatr Orthop 4:246, 1984.

Staheli LT: Femoral and tibial growth following femoral shaft fracture in childhood. Clin Orthop 55:159, 1967.

Wagner H: Operative lengthening of the femur. Clin Orthop 136:125, 1978.

Hemihypertrophy and Hemiatrophy

Letts RM: Orthopaedic treatment of hemangiomatous hypertrophy of the lower extremity. J Bone Joint Surg 59A:777, 1977.

MacEwen GD and Case JL: Congenital hemihypertrophy. A review of 32 cases. Clin Orthop 50:147, 1967.

Specht EE and Hazelrig PE: Orthopaedic considerations of Silver's syndrome. J Bone Joint Surg 55A:1502, 1973.

Patellofemoral Problems

Casscells SW: Chondromalacia of the patella. J Pediatr Orthop 2:560, 1982.

Crosby EB and Insall J: Recurrent dislocation of the patella. J Bone Joint Surg 58A:9, 1976.

Ficat RP and Hungerford DS: Disorders of the Patellofemoral Joint. Baltimore, Williams & Wilkins Co., 1977.

Goodfellow J et al.: Patellofemoral joint mechanics and pathology. J Bone Joint Surg 58B:291, 1976.

Gruber MA: The conservative treatment of chondromalacia patella. Orthop Clin North Am 10:105, 1979.

Hughston JC: Subluxation of the patella. J Bone Joint Surg 50A:1003, 1968.

Insall J et al.: Chondromalacia patellae: A prospective study. J Bone Joint Surg 58A:1, 1976.

Internal Knee Problems

Kaplan EB: Discoid lateral meniscus of the knee joint. Nature, mechanism and operative treatment. J Bone Joint Surg 39A:77, 1957.

Osteochondritis Dissecans

Green WT and Banks HH: Osteochondritis dissecans in children. J Bone Joint Surg 35A:26, 1953.

Linden B: Osteochondritis dissecans of the femoral condyles. A longterm follow-up study. J Bone Joint Surg 59A:769, 1977.

Zeman SC and Nelson MW: Osteochondritis dissecans of the knee. Orthop Rev 7–9:101, 1978.

Osgood-Schlatter Disease

Mital MA et al.: The so-called unresolved Osgood-Schlatter lesion. J Bone Joint Surg 62A:732, 1980.

Ogden JA and Southwick WO: Osgood-Schlatter's disease and tibial tuberosity development. Clin Orthop 116:180, 1976.

Willner P: Osgood-Schlatter disease. Etiology and treatment. Clin Orthop 62:178, 1969.

Popliteal Cyst

Dinham JM: Popliteal cysts in children: The case against surgery. J Bone Joint Surg 57B:69, 1975.

MacMahon EB: Baker's cysts in children: Is surgery necessary? J Bone Joint Surg 55A:1311, 1973.

Osteomyelitis

Fox L and Sprunt K: Neonatal osteomyelitis. Pediatrics 62:535, 1978.

Morrey BF and Peterson HA: Hematogenous pyogenic osteomyelitis in children. Orthop Clin North Am 6:935, 1975.

Tetzlaff TR et al.: Oral antibiotic therapy for skeletal infections in children. J Pediatr 92:485, 1978.

Trueta J: The three types of acute haematogenous osteomyelitis. A clinical and vascular study. J Bone Joint Surg 41B:671, 1959.

Waldvogel FA and Vasey H: Osteomyelitis: The past decade. N Engl J Med 303:360, 1980.

Septic Arthritis

Curtiss PH Jr: Bone and joint infections in childhood. American Academy of Orthopaedic Surgeons Instructional Course Lectures 26:14, 1977.

Morrey BF et al.: Septic arthritis in children. Orthop Clin North Am 6:923, 1975.

Leg Pains

Apley J: Limb pains with no organic disease. Clin Rheum Dis 2:487, 1976.

Oster J: Recurrent abdominal pain, headache, and limb pains in children and adolescents. Pediatrics 50:429, 1972.

Oster J and Nielsen A: Growing pains: A clinical justification of a school population. Acta Pediatr Scand 61:329, 1972.

Peterson HA: Leg aches. Pediatr Clin North Am 24:731, 1977.

Trauma

Blount WP: Fractures in Children. Baltimore, Williams & Wilkins Co., 1955.

Rang M: Children's Fractures. Philadelphia, JB Lippincott Co, 1974.

Salter RB and Harris WR: Injuries involving the epiphyseal plate. J Bone Joint Surg 45A:587, 1963.

6

The Foot

Apparent and real variations in the structure and function of the foot are exceedingly common in children. They often cause considerable confusion and anxiety on the part of parents, grandparents, and other family members.

INTOEING

Intoeing is the most common reason for taking a child to a health care practitioner for treatment of perceived lower extremity problems. This subject has been partially addressed in Chapter 5, in which femoral anteversion and internal tibial torsion were discussed.

The cause of intoeing can often be accurately guessed simply by knowing the age of the child. In newborns, it is most likely to be caused by either metatarsus varus or clubfoot. These are readily apparent in the newborn nursery. Later on in infancy, other causes, such as overactivity of the abductor hallucis, dynamic intoeing, and internal tibial torsion, are often the reason. In the young child, either internal tibial torsion or medial deviation of the talar neck is most likely to be the cause, since other intrinsic foot problems usually will have been corrected before walking age. Femoral anteversion is the most common cause in older children, being noted when a gait pattern has been established.

Metatarsus Varus (Metatarsus Adductus)

Metatarsus varus is the most common congenital foot deformity, occurring once per thousand births. It may be related to intrauterine positioning. The incidence of one per thousand increases to about five per cent with subsequent pregnancies, indicating that there may be familial factors as well. In some series, males are affected more commonly than females, whereas in others the reverse is true. An association with congenital dysplasia of the hip has been reported in 5% to 10% of patients.

The clinical presentation is a varus and mild supination deviation at the tarsometatarsal joints, most prominently at the first joint. It decreases in severity from a medial direction to a lateral one (Fig. 6–1). The normally straight or slightly convex lateral border of the foot has an exaggerated convexity in metatarsus varus, such that the fifth metatarsal may be subject to excessive weight-bearing forces. The hindfoot is usually neutral or in slight valgus. Internal tibial torsion is commonly seen.

The treatment of metatarsus varus depends upon its severity at the time of diagnosis. Many feet are supple and passively overcorrectable without difficulty. For such feet, no treatment or, at most, simple stretching exercises may be prescribed, to be done by the parents at the time of diaper changes. These consist of holding the heel firmly in one hand and gently exerting corrective pressure against the first metatarsal with the other. Stretching exercises should be used with caution, since parents may not perform them properly, and with improper stretching there is a risk of increasing the heel valgus and producing a flat foot. If the child habitually sits or sleeps with the feet tucked under the buttocks, then it may be advisable to use

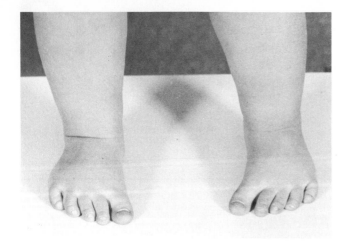

Figure 6–1. Bilateral metatarsus varus.

straight-last or outflare shoes to prevent the forces of gravity, the pelvis, and the upper body from perpetuating the deformity. The shoes are often prescribed to be worn day and night, except to attend to foot hygiene, until the condition has resolved.

If the foot is not passively correctable, then serial manipulation and use of a plaster cast at intervals of every week or two will produce correction. A below-knee cast is usually sufficient, although with abnormal internal tibial torsion, an above-knee cast with the knee in flexion is more corrective. Treatment is continued until the foot is passively overcorrectable, which usually takes no more than one or two months. Then use of holding casts or of straight-last or outflare shoes is appropriate until there is no tendency for recurrence. Serial casting is always effective before the age of one year, usually effective between the ages of one and two years, and rarely effective when rigid metatarsus varus persists after the age of two years. The older child will require surgical release of the tarsometatarsal joints or, if older than the age of six years, metatarsal osteotomies.

It is worthy to note that when all cases of metatarsus varus are considered together, approximately 85% will resolve spontaneously without any treatment. Most of these are in the passively overcorrectable group at the time of diagnosis. The ultimate result of the foot with untreated, rigid metatarsus varus is pain, caused by excessive weight-bearing over the lateral border of the foot, and substantial difficulty in obtaining adequate footwear.

Clubfoot (Talipes Equinovarus)

Talipes equinovarus is a complex foot deformity that is readily apparent at birth. It is characterized by an equinus positioning of the entire foot with pronounced varus of the heel and even further varus and supination of the forefoot (Fig. 6–2). The incidence of clubfoot is slightly less than one per thousand, although it is much higher if there is a positive family history. The male-to-female ratio is two to one, and bilaterality is common.

The cause of clubfoot is unknown, but it may be a multifactorial condition for which one would have a genetic predisposition. Intrauterine factors and oligohydramnios may also play a role in some, but not all, cases. There is good evidence that neuromuscular involvement is one primary factor in its de-

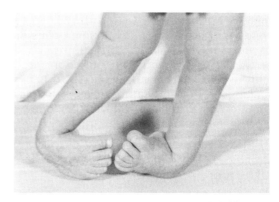

Figure 6–2. Bilateral severe congenital clubfeet.

velopment (Handelsman and Badalemente). Clubfoot also occurs with many neurologic conditions, such as myelomeningocele, sacral agenesis, and arthrogryposis mutiplex congenita.

Radiologic findings in clubfoot are characteristic, but care must be taken to position the foot properly for the films. In the infant, the talus and the calcaneus are the only ossified tarsal bones. Normally, they are oriented at about a 30-degree angle in both anteroposterior (AP) and lateral views. Their parallelism in both views is a pathognomonic diagnostic feature (Fig. 6–3). Varus of the metatarsals is also easily recognizable.

There are variations in the severity of clubfeet. Some are relatively flexible and are correctable with serial manipulations and casting. The earlier that nonsurgical treatment is begun, the more likely it is to be successful. Treatment can often be initiated in the newborn nursery and should consist of gentle manipulative correction applied in a sequential fashion. One should not attempt to correct all components of the deformity at once. The forefoot varus is corrected first, then the hindfoot varus, and finally the equinus. If this sequence is not followed, a rocker-bottom foot deformity will result. Manipulation must be gentle and careful to prevent damage to the cartilaginous tarsal anlagen. Manipulation is followed by either plaster cast application or taping, and it should be repeated at intervals of one to two days. After the first week or two, weekly changes are satisfactory. If it is apparent on clinical and radiographic examination that correction has not been achieved in three to six months, then surgical treatment should be strongly considered.

It is very important that families understand that a clubfoot will never be a normal foot. Some deformity will persist, and the leg will always be smaller. Nevertheless, with appropriate treatment, function may be restored to nearly normal.

For those feet with more moderate or severe involvement, the best results come from surgical treatment. In many cases, even after surgical correction, prolonged orthotic control of the foot and ankle is necessary to insure a maximally good result. Use of night splints is frequently necessary to prevent recurrent equinus of the heel.

The standard of surgical care consists of a one-stage soft tissue release that allows realignment of the bones, followed by internal fixation and maintenance of the correction in casts for several months. The timing of surgery depends upon the severity of the

Figure 6–3. *A,* Radiographs of clubfoot show parallelism of the talus and calcaneus. Equinus of the calcaneus is seen on a lateral radiograph. *B,* The AP radiograph of the same foot shows parallelism of the talus and calcaneus, and varus angulation of the metatarsals compared with the hindfoot.

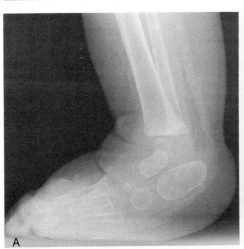
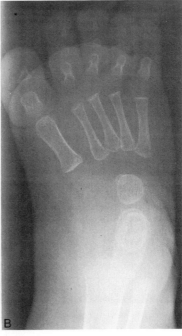

clubfoot, the size of the child, and the experience of the surgeon. In the majority of cases, it is best to operate on patients between the ages of 3 and 18 months.

Abductor Hallucis Overactivity

In this self-explanatory condition, the abductor hallucis muscle, which originates on the medial side of the calcaneus and inserts on the medial side of the proximal phalanx of the great toe, appears overactive compared with the adductor and produces the so-called "searching big toe" (Fig. 6–4). The great toe (and sometimes the entire forefoot distal to the tarsometatarsal joints) is pulled into varus. This is most often noted early in infancy and is best treated by reassurance of the parents. It does not interfere with shoe fitting and usually disappears by the age of one or two years. Less than one per cent of cases will show persistent activity into early childhood. If it persists past the age of three years, tendon lengthening or surgical release should be considered.

Dynamic Intoeing

During infancy, most children have a strong plantar grasp reflex with toe flexion, forefoot supination, and adduction. This gives the appearance of intoeing, but when the child is examined passively there is no fixed deformity such as metatarsus varus,

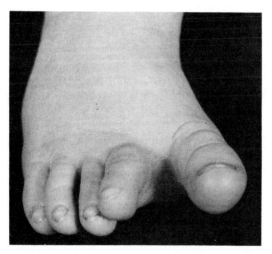

Figure 6–4. Abductor hallucis overactivity (searching big toe).

clubfoot, excessive internal tibial torsion, or excessive femoral anteversion. The intoeing may persist after the child begins walking, but again, on examination nothing pathologic is detected. In such cases, gradual resolution of the inward-deviating angle of the gait is the rule, and reassurance is all that is necessary. This is predicated on the fact that one has ruled out muscle imbalance secondary to such conditions as cerebral palsy or other neuromuscular diseases. In cases of idiopathic dynamic intoeing, there may be a positive family history. It is good to tell parents that a few more years of growth and development may be required before the condition disappears, and that at times the amount of intoeing may even appear to be increasing. Remind them that adult gait patterns do not develop until the age of four or five years. It should be made clear that shoe modifications in any form will not affect this type of intoeing.

Medial Deviation of the Talar Neck

Particularly in children younger than the age of six years, medial deviation of the talar neck has been identified by Bleck as a cause of intoeing. This exceedingly rare condition is characterized by normal tibiofibular torsion but internal axial deviation of the foot from the midsagittal plane. Its cause is persistence of the fetal medial deviation of the neck of the talus.

According to Bleck, in children younger than three years old, spontaneous correction with growth occurs if the feet are deviated inward 10 degrees or less. If more than 10 degrees of deviation is found, then a Denis Browne splint is used up to the age of 18 months, and a twister cable orthosis is occasionally effective after the age of three years. After six years of age, significantly deformed feet will require surgical treatment by means of a wedge osteotomy.

FLAT FEET

Children are frequently referred to the physician for evaluation of flat feet. The issue is to determine whether the flat feet are a normal physiologic variation or a pathologic condition. The normal infant has a fat foot, which gives the illusion of being flat. If one were to take footprints serially from birth to early childhood, one would see a progressive decrease in the width of the midfoot as growth proceeds. The normal longitudinal arch of the foot usually develops by the age of five years.

Physiologic Flatfoot

The most common flatfoot is the flexible physiologic type, which is often seen in families and occurs more commonly in Jewish and black people than in the overall population. These feet are easily detectable because they are mobile, have excellent muscle strength, and are uniformly painless, unless the deformity is severe. These patients present with loss of the normal medial longitudinal arch of the foot (Fig. 6–5). During weightbearing, the heel appears to be in slightly increased valgus. When the child stands on tiptoes, the arch is restored, and the heel is neutral or tends to go into slight varus. With further growth, ligamentous laxity will decrease, and the diminution of baby fat also accounts for some improvement. In the past, a commonly held myth has been that flat feet are weak feet, and that they can be corrected by such exercises as picking up objects with the toes. This is false. In fact, intrinsic foot muscle weakness or paralysis leads to a high arch or cavus foot. Conditions such as femoral anteversion, genu valgus, and other problems with increased ligamentous laxity may also be associated with flexible flat feet.

Radiographs taken of the foot while bearing weight show flattening of the arch and an increase in the talocalcaneal angle, in both the AP and the lateral projections, as the talus becomes more vertical because of less support from the valgus calcaneus. Ordinarily, radiographs do not need to be obtained when the feet are flexible and painless. It is rare for such feet ever to become symptomatic.

Treatment may be indicated for the more severe varieties of hypermobile flat feet, either to prolong shoe wear (with full knowledge that one is treating the shoes and not the feet), to prevent ligaments from being overstretched, or for relief in those cases in which there are mild symptoms of fatigue or discomfort with increased activity. In these cases, the usual prescription is to place a one-eighth-inch medial heel wedge and a navicular pad (arch support) in a firm, oxford-type shoe with good support in the lateral and medial heel areas. This is the so-called "orthopedic shoe." It should be remembered that this will not correct the foot in any way but will simply prolong the shoe wear, prevent ligament overstretching, or relieve mild symptoms. For patients with extremely severe hypermobile flatfoot, more formal shoe orthotics may be necessary. These are very expensive and require frequent changing during growth. Although several surgical procedures have been devised in attempts to correct hypermobile flat feet, the only indications for surgery are severe uncorrectable deformity or pain not relieved by use of appropriate foot orthotics.

There is an entity known as "hypermobile flatfoot with short tendo-Achilles" (Harris and Beath). This has the clinical appearance

Figure 6–5. A typical flexible flatfoot with a valgus heel and flat longitudinal arch.

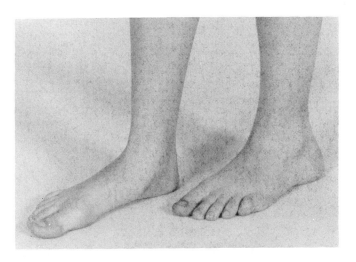

of a flexible flatfoot, but dorsiflexion of the foot is significantly limited. It often responds to heel-cord stretching exercises.

Pathologic Flatfoot

Pathologic pes planus, or rigid flatfoot, is commonly seen in conjunction with neuromuscular diseases, tarsal coalition, infection in the foot, juvenile rheumatoid arthritis, or a bone cyst or a tumor in the foot.

Tarsal Coalition

The most common nonneuromuscular cause of pathologic flatfoot is tarsal coalition, whereby two or more of the tarsal bones are united either by a bony bar or by a fibrocartilaginous bridge (Fig. 6–6). The result is a rigid flatfoot, occasionally associated with spasm of the peroneal musculature. The cause of the coalition is probably incomplete separation of the mesenchymal anlagen of the tarsal bones. The bar may be fibrous or cartilaginous at first and may then ossify during further growth. The most common locations for the bar are the calcaneonavicular area and the talocalcaneal coalition. Much less common are talonavicular and calcaneo-

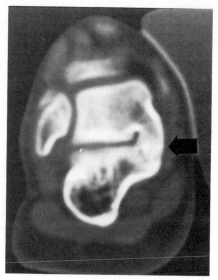

Figure 6–7. Computerized tomogram demonstrating coalition of the middle talocalcaneal facet.

cuboid bars. Rarely, more than one coalition will exist in the same foot. Bilaterality is common. There is often an autosomal dominant inheritance pattern.

The pathologic effect of the coalition is to decrease motion markedly in the hindfoot, particularly pronation and supination around the long axis of the foot. These are needed for smoothing out gait when walking on uneven terrain. It is postulated that the coalition causes increased stress at other tarsal joints and subsequent early degenerative arthritis, particularly in the talonavicular joint. This is consistent with the observation that most people with coalitions do not become symptomatic until late childhood or adolescence, although many coalitions never become symptomatic.

When a painful, rigid foot is seen, appropriate radiographs need to be obtained to confirm the diagnosis. The calcaneonavicular bar is best detected on an oblique view of the hindfoot. Talocalcaneal coalition is sometimes seen on the plain lateral view, but usually either computerized tomography or special angulated axial projections are required (Fig. 6–7). An ordinary AP radiograph is sufficient to detect the talonavicular and calcaneocuboid coalitions.

Conservative treatment by means of shoe modifications, restriction of activities, use of nonsteroidal medications, foot orthotics, or manipulation and temporary immobilization in a plaster cast may be tried, but they rarely

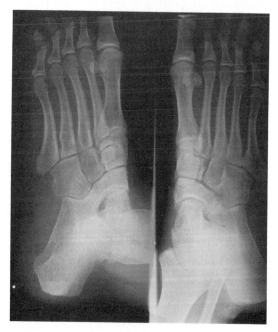

Figure 6–6. Bilateral calcaneonavicular coalition—complete on the left, incomplete on the right.

produce lasting relief. Recalcitrant painful feet require surgical treatment. In cases in which there are no significant degenerative changes and the patient is not yet skeletally mature, excision of the bar with free fat-graft interposition to prevent reossification is usually successful. Other coalitions, particularly those associated with degenerative changes, require the triple arthrodesis procedure for relief of pain.

Calcaneovalgus

This type of supple, nonrigid flatfoot presents with the calcaneus dorsiflexed and the foot pronated. Calcaneovalgus will always accompany the entity known as "posteromedial bowing of the tibia" and may be associated with congenital hip dysplasia, but more commonly it occurs as an isolated event, probably as the result of aberrant intrauterine posi-

tioning. When seen shortly after birth, the foot usually will not plantarflex to neutral, and the heel is in moderate valgus. On radiographic examination, this condition is differentiated from a congenital vertical talus by the fact that the hindfoot is in dorsiflexion, not plantar flexion (Fig. 6–8). Calcaneovalgus is easily managed with stretching exercises followed by taping or immobilization in a cast, if needed.

Convex Pes Valgus (Vertical Talus)

This is a congenital condition that presents at birth as a severe flatfoot or rocker-bottom foot. Radiographic evaluation demonstrates the talus to be in a vertical position, the navicular anlage being dislocated onto its dorsal surface (Fig. 6–8). The calcaneus is in equinus. The cause of the vertical talus is unknown. It is frequently associated with

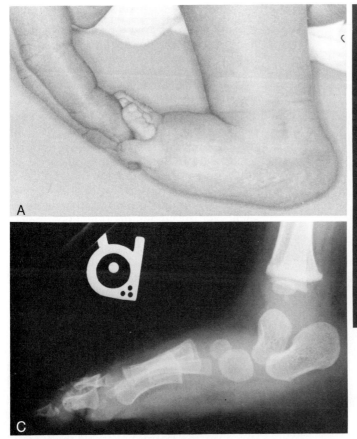
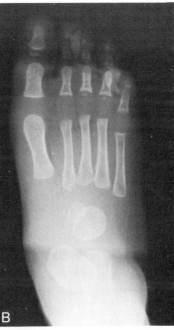

Figure 6–8. *A,* Congenital convex pes valgus. The foot appears dorsiflexed, but the calcaneus is actually in equinus, and the talus is in a vertical position. AP *(B)* and lateral *(C)* radiographs of congenital convex pes valgus. Note the vertical position of the talus and the equinus attitude of the calcaneus on the lateral view.

other neuromuscular disease. This condition is easily differentiated from other forms of flatfoot by its rigidity and its radiographic appearance.

The initial treatment of convex pes valgus may consist of stretching of the mid- and forefoot in an attempt to reduce it into an equinus position and line it up with the nearly vertical hindfoot. If this is possible, then later the entire foot may be dorsiflexed as a unit. Nonsurgical treatment is rarely successful, however, and the foot usually requires extensive surgical release for correction of the deformity. This is a complex and difficult operation but can produce excellent and durable results. It should be done before the age of three years. The natural history of the untreated congenital vertical talus is foot pain, rigidity, and interference with walking.

TOE WALKERS

Some children begin walking with a toe–toe type of gait instead of the normal heel–toe weight-bearing progression (Fig. 6–9). These children walk with metatarsal-head weight-bearing from the onset of ambulation.

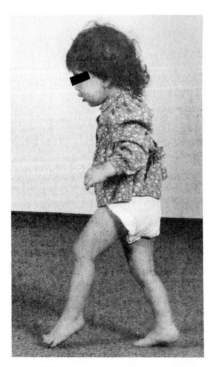

Figure 6–9. This two-year-old girl is an idiopathic toe walker.

The condition is twice as common in boys, and in approximately one third of the cases, there is a family history of toe walking. There is no pain or limitation of activity. Toe walking can be caused by cerebral palsy or other neuromuscular conditions. These being ruled out, the child belongs in the category of the true "idiopathic toe walker." These children tend to be more clumsy than their peers and also are often more hyperactive.

It is important to determine whether there is a coexisting heel cord contracture, which occurs in half the cases. Those with no tightness of the heel cord are able to stand voluntarily with a plantigrade foot and can consciously walk with a normal heel–toe gait, but they usually walk on their toes. In these cases, reassurance is the treatment. Resolution will occur sometime during childhood.

If a tight heel cord is present, then stretching exercises may be successful, although serial or "drop-out" cast correction is more definitive. Those with tight heel cords are more likely to have a family history of the condition. If recurrence is noted, a search for a neurologic cause is appropriate. The only indication for surgical elongation of the heel cord and release of the posterior ankle capsule is progressive or resistant tightness. This is present in fewer than one per cent of true idiopathic toewalkers.

CAVUS FOOT

A cavus deformity of the foot is a high medial longitudinal plantar arch, usually associated with dorsiflexion of the calcaneus and with equinus, supination, and varus deviation of the forefoot (Fig. 6–10). It is most commonly found in neuromuscular diseases such as myelomeningocele, poliomyelitis, Friedreich's ataxia, Charcot-Marie-Tooth disease (hereditary motor and sensory neuropathy), and intraspinal tumors. A much less common and often familial condition is the idiopathic cavus or cavovarus foot.

The idiopathic type of deformity is usually only a cosmetic deformity in young children, but it tends to increase during growth and become symptomatic in adolescence or adult life. The symptom to note is pain in the longitudinal arch and lateral border of the foot, which probably is secondary to chronic ligamentous strain and maldistribution of weight-bearing forces with increased pressure over the lateral border of the foot. The

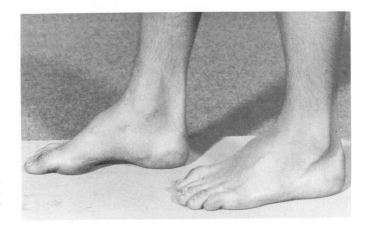

Figure 6–10. Bilateral cavovarus feet. Note the high arch. Patients with this deformity should be suspected of having a lower spinal lesion.

approach to this condition is to search first for a neurologic cause and manage that appropriately. The specific treatment of cavus foot depends upon the age of the patient. Children may respond to soft tissue releases and corrective casting, although osteotomy of the calcaneus is also frequently necessary. Adults will require osteotomy through the midfoot or a triple arthrodesis for correction.

FOOT PAIN

Metatarsalgia

Older children with one or more unusually prominent metatarsal heads in the plantar aspect of their feet, often associated with mild cavus, will frequently complain of pain in the distal metatarsal region. The discomfort may be relieved by use of pads or bars placed transversely across the shoe, either on the sole or as an insert, just proximal to the metatarsal heads. When metatarsalgia is severe and recalcitrant, consideration of metatarsal osteotomy should be given. This procedure almost always provides lasting relief.

Stress Fractures

Older children and adolescents who subject their feet to prolonged walking or running may develop stress fractures, commonly seen as transverse fractures of the metatarsal shafts (Fig. 6–11). These are most common in the second and third metatarsals, although in conditions in which there is uncorrected forefoot varus, the fifth metatarsal may be the site. Stress fractures may be extremely difficult to detect on radiographic examination in their early stages. They usually present as localized pain over the metatarsal, which is tender to palpation. Weight-bearing increases the pain. Bone scans show localized increased uptake and are usually diagnostic. Many cases will present with the radiographic appearance of a healing fracture.

Treatment consists of restricting activities,

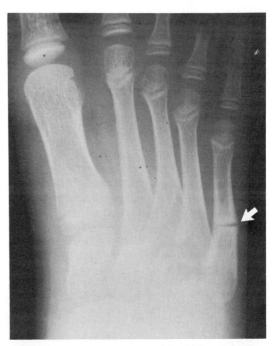

Figure 6–11. Stress fracture of the fifth metatarsal.

although in more severe cases use of a walking cast may be appropriate.

Plantar Fascia Pain

This presents as pain and tenderness over the plantar fascia, particularly at its origin on the anterior calcaneus, but also may occur along the medial longitudinal arch of the foot. It can be idiopathic or can be caused by overuse, such as running or jumping, or by isolated trauma. It may also be associated with fibromatosis of the plantar fascia. Mild cavus deformity is a frequent finding.

Treatment consists of conservative measures, including restriction of activities, use of a one-quarter-inch padded heel lift inside the shoe, use of soft molded shoe inserts or arch supports, or physical therapy modalities such as heat, massage, ultrasound, or other techniques. Surgical excision of painful plantar fibromatosis may be required. Although steroid injections and surgical release of the painful plantar fascia have been advocated, the results are often disappointing.

Freiberg's Infraction

Avascular necrosis of the head of a metatarsal bone is known as Freiberg's infraction (Fig. 6–12). It most often involves the second metatarsal because it is the longest and most rigid, but the infraction can occur in the third and fourth as well. Girls are afflicted more often than boys, usually during adolescence. Its presentation is one of pain and tenderness, without swelling, over the involved metatarsal, and it often produces a noticeable limp. The radiographic picture is typical for avascular necrosis—sclerosis, irregularity, and some collapse of the metatarsal head. Repeated trauma may play a role in its development, and occasionally a concomitant stress fracture of the metatarsal shaft is seen.

Treatment is symptomatic and consists of restriction of activities, use of a metatarsal pad in the shoe or a metatarsal bar on the sole proximal to the lesion, or application of a short-leg walking cast. If pain is more severe, relief from weight-bearing is appropriate. The vast majority of cases are self limited and will ultimately revascularize, leaving the metatarsal head minimally deformed but restoring full function.

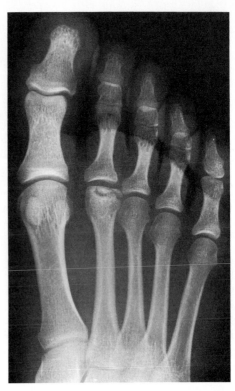

Figure 6–12. Freiberg's infraction of the second metatarsal head.

Köhler's Disease

This condition is analogous to Freiberg's infraction and represents avascular necrosis of the tarsal navicular bone. About 80% of cases occur in boys, and the age of onset is usually between four and seven years of age. The clinical picture is one of pain, tenderness, occasional local swelling, and often a noticeable limp. Bilateral disease occurs in 25% of the patients. The cause is unknown, but, again, recurrent mild trauma may be implicated. Mild cases may be difficult to diagnose on radiographic examination, since the tarsal navicular bone normally often develops in an irregular fashion. The usual radiographic picture of Köhler's disease shows increased sclerosis with flattening, irregularity, and fragmentation of the navicular bone (Fig. 6–13). Comparison views of the asymptomatic opposite foot may be helpful.

Appropriate treatment is conservative. Restricting activities for a brief period of time is usually all that is necessary. Should symptoms persist, immobilization three to four weeks in a short-leg walking cast is helpful.

Kidner's Disease (Tarsal Navicular Bursitis)

In this condition, an accessory ossicle medial to the tarsal navicular may be present, as it is in 12% of the population, or a large hypertrophic medial projection of the tarsal navicular bone may be seen (Fig. 6–14). This can become painful owing to either overlying bursitis or strain of the attachment of the posterior tibial tendon at that point. Treatment consists of restriction of activities. If this is unsuccessful, a one-fourth-inch heel lift or one-eight-inch medial heel wedge, or both, may be tried. If relief is still not attained, a local steroid injection may be helpful. The next step in conservative care is three to four weeks of immobilization in a short-leg walking cast. Should all else fail (which is extremely rare) and the condition becomes chronic and severe, surgical excision of the offending bone may be necessary.

Sever's Disease

Sever's disease causes pain, which increases with exercise, over the posterior surface of the calcaneus. It usually occurs in children between the ages of 6 and 12 years. The

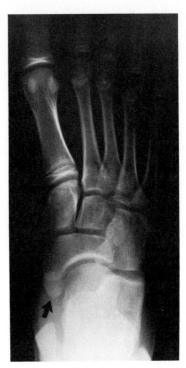

Figure 6–14. Accessory tarsal navicular-bone.

pathologic mechanism is probably a chronic strain at the insertion of the Achilles tendon. Radiographs show increased density and fragmentation of the calcaneal apophysis, but this is, in fact, always a normal radiographic finding for this multicentric ossification center. A comparison view will readily substantiate this. The condition is self limited, although some reduction in activity may be advisable. A slight heel lift is also helpful. If this fails, three to four weeks' use of a short-leg walking cast should resolve the problem.

Other Heel Pain

Pain directly over the plantar surface of the calcaneus may be caused by chronic stress at the origin of the plantar fascia or by chronic minor trauma secondary to overuse, such as recently increased walking or other activities involving repeated heel strikes. Also, it may be secondary to bone lesions of the calcaneus, for example a benign bone cyst, osteomyelitis, osteoid osteoma, or another tumor (Fig. 6–15). In cases for which no apparent cause can be found, treatment is conservative, consisting of either the wearing of a soft, cushioned-heel type of shoe, or,

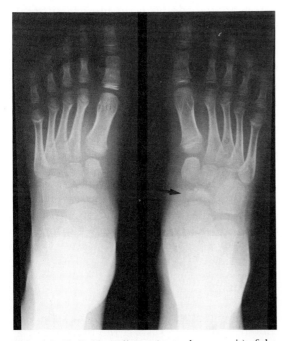

Figure 6–13. Köhler's disease (avascular necrosis) of the right tarsal navicular bone.

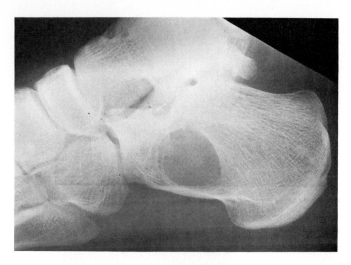

Figure 6–15. A unicameral bone cyst of the calcaneus. This patient presented with heel pain.

if this fails, (paradoxically) the use of a firm plastic heel cup inside the shoe.

Pump Bumps

These are painful prominences just above the insertion of the Achilles tendon at the superior posterior margin of the calcaneus. They are usually bilateral. Although often thought to be caused by chronic friction from rubbing against the upper edge of the shoe, they more often arise spontaneously, either as a form of retro-Achilles tendon inflammation or as an unusual prominence of the posterior calcaneus on an idiopathic basis. The condition is managed by avoiding restrictive or friction-producing footwear. For chronically enlarged and painful lesions, surgical excision is curative.

Plantar Warts

Plantar wart lesions occur singly or in clusters in any area of the plantar skin and are most painful when they occur in the major weight-bearing areas. Treatment consists of purchasing an inexpensive kit, over-the-counter, in any drug store. The kit contains salicylic acid in collodion, which is painted on the wart twice a day and subsequently covered with a bandage. Using a felt or moleskin pad or donut to relieve weight-bearing over the painful wart may also be helpful. Softening and atrophy of the wart then occur over a period of several days to several months. This is highly effective in the vast majority of cases. More aggressive treatment, such as cauterization, freezing, enucleation, or surgical excision, should be a last resort and, if necessary, should be done carefully in order to avoid producing a painful scar.

TOE PROBLEMS

Syndactyly

Syndactyly of the toes may be complete or incomplete. This is a cosmetic problem only. Unless another deformity is present, surgical treatment is not usually indicated.

Polydactyly

The significance of polydactyly in the foot is to alert the examiner to look for other congenital anomalies in the lower or upper limbs. Small hypoplastic accessory toes should be removed early, but with larger anomalies, it is best to wait until function and bony anatomy can be assessed. Usually by the age of two years, an appropriate decision can be made regarding the proper ablation needed to narrow the foot and to allow satisfactory shoe fitting.

Macrodactyly

Local gigantism or enlargement of a toe should lead one to suspect the presence of a vascular anomaly or neurofibromatosis. Treatment can be deferred until there is

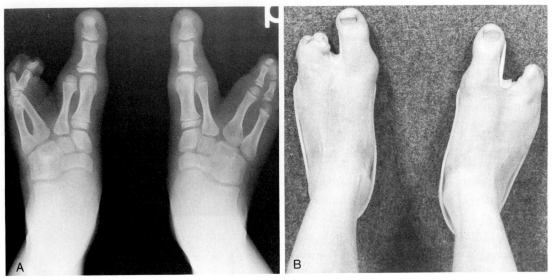

Figure 6–16. *A,* Bilateral ectrodactyly of the feet. *B,* The same patient after surgery to narrow the foot and facilitate shoe fitting.

interference with shoe fitting or until there is a negative psychologic impact on the child. Then a procedure such as amputation or reduction by means of bone and soft tissue resection may be appropriate.

Ectrodactyly (Lobster-Claw Foot)

This condition is usually inherited on an autosomal dominant basis and may be associated with ectrodactyly of the hand and other congenital anomalies, such as cleft lip, cleft palate, or deafness. It is a major cosmetic deformity but rarely interferes with function and responds quite well to surgical narrowing of the foot (Fig. 6–16). Although a normal foot cannot be produced, significant improvement is the rule, and this may be of great psychologic benefit to the child.

Overlapping Toes

The curling-under or overlapping of toes may be a familial condition, probably caused by abnormalities of the toe bones or of the intrinsic muscles of the feet. One fourth of these may be expected to improve with growth and not require treatment.

Overlapping of toes is usually an isolated condition. It is most often bilateral and asymptomatic (Fig. 6–17). Before the age of one year, treatment is unnecessary. Later,

when the foot is of sufficient size, one may consider taping the toes in a corrected position, with absorbable cotton placed in the web space. Although taping is rarely curative, it does buy time and allow for further growth to make surgery simpler. Use of accommodative footwear is the best means of treating the symptomatic overlapping toe in a young child. If symptoms develop owing to shoe friction, surgical correction may be required. This is best deferred until after the age of

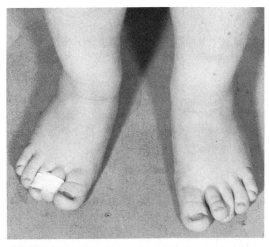

Figure 6–17. Bilateral overlapping toes illustrate temporizing and usually unsuccessful treatment of the right foot.

three years, when the toes are larger. The corrective surgery involves tendon lengthening or transfer or, if deferred until adolescence, arthrodesis of the appropriate toe joint.

Hammer Toes and Claw Toes

A hammer toe is a flexion contracture of the proximal interphalangeal (PIP) joint with hyperextension at the metatarsophalangeal joint. The distal joint may be normal or in flexion contracture. The deformity is most common in the second toe but is also seen in the third and fourth toes. Hammer toes, as distinct from claw toes, are isolated findings and may be bilateral. The patient presents with pain caused by bursitis and chronic friction over the dorsum of the PIP joint and, less commonly, over the plantar aspect of the metatarsal head. If the wearing of accommodative footwear with an adequate toe box is unsuccessful, then the best treatment is arthrodesis of the proximal joint in a straight position, with soft tissue release and tendon lengthening at the metatarsophalangeal joint, if needed. In severe cases, an osteotomy of the metatarsal may also be necessary.

A claw toe deformity is a neurologic condition, usually accompanied by pes cavus and intrinsic muscle atrophy. Clawing of the toes is a deformity similar to hammer toes, with metatarsophalangeal extension and interphalangeal flexion. Common causative conditions are myelomeningocele, polio, degenerative neuromuscular diseases, cerebral palsy, and lesions of the caudal spinal cord and nerve roots. Neurologic and electromyographic studies show involvement of the intrinsic muscles of the foot. Treatment is then directed at the underlying cause. The cavus foot and claw toes usually require surgical treatment, the specifics of which depend upon the age of the patient and the severity of the foot deformity.

Hallux Valgus (Bunion)

This condition, extremely common in adults, is rarely seen in young children but may be noted in preadolescents or adolescents. Most cases are probably caused by congenital or developmental abnormalities in the first ray, particularly the first cuneiform

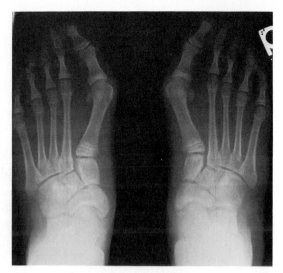

Figure 6–18. Bilateral hallux valgus deformity with excessive varus of the first metatarsal bilaterally.

and metatarsal regions (Fig. 6–18). Varus deviation of the first ray is the pathologic disorder in most cases, with subsequent adaptive valgus angulation at the metatarsophalangeal joint secondary to the soft-tissue bowstringing or muscle imbalance with overpulling of the adductor hallucis. A pointed-toe or ill-fitting shoe may exacerbate the deformity but is not the sole cause, since hallux valgus is also found in people who have never worn shoes. The significance of hallux valgus, other than its cosmetic deformity, is the occurrence of painful bursitis over the medial aspect of the head of the first metatarsal. Usually, the pain is relieved by wearing shoes with a wide toe box. Unless extremely severe, the deformity does not interfere with great toe function during walking.

Surgical correction of hallux valgus may be accomplished by a variety of means and should be individualized according to the age of the patient and the disorder present. The indications for surgery are significant cosmetic deformity, problems with shoe fitting, or recurrent pain from the bursitis over the bunion. In children, the procedure of choice is an osteotomy of the first metatarsal bone.

An analogous condition, when present in the fifth ray with discomfort over the lateral head of the fifth metatarsal, is called a "bunionette" (Fig. 6–19). It is managed, in principle, similarly to hallux valgus.

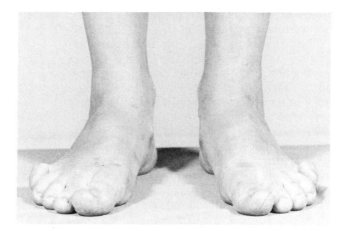

Figure 6–19. Bilateral bunionette deformities.

Uncus Incarnatus (Ingrown Toenail)

This painful lesion is caused by the overgrowth of the edge of the toenail in a lateral and plantar direction. The ingrowing nail is an irritant and causes an inflammatory response, frequently with an associated bacterial infection and hypertrophic granulation tissue. Mild cases respond to warm soaks and gentle elevation of the involved side of the toenail by careful packing with absorbent cotton until the condition has resolved. More advanced cases require excision of the lateral side of the toenail with the patient under local anesthesia. The nail usually grows back in a more appropriate position, although the recurrence rate is high. Severe cases require excision of the lateral half of the nail, curettage of the nail bed, and excision of the granulation and other soft tissue. Instruction in proper cutting of the toenails—in a transverse fashion as opposed to rounded—is important.

FRACTURES OF THE FOOT AND THE TOES

Fractures of the feet of children are very uncommon before adolescence, when they are usually caused by high-velocity injuries involving motorcycles or automobiles. Fractures of the toes are usually the result of blunt trauma, such as kicking an inanimate object or having the toes caught in a door or in bicycle spokes. Most fractures are either nondisplaced or minimally displaced and are best treated by taping the involved toe to an adjacent one, with cotton interposed in the web space. This should be maintained for two to three weeks or until symptoms disappear. Displaced phalangeal fractures require reduction using a local anesthetic block. If unstable, pin fixation and a plaster cast may be necessary.

Metatarsal fractures may be stress fractures or may result from blunt trauma. Displacement is usually absent or minimal, and three to four weeks in a short-leg walking cast is adequate treatment.

Tarsal bone fractures are very different in children. They usually are the result of jumping from a great height. If nondisplaced, they are managed by use of a compression dressing or an extremely well-padded cast and crutches, with the involved limb in a onweight-bearing position for three to six weeks. Displaced tarsal bone fractures should be openly reduced if closed reduction is not perfect.

CHILDREN'S SHOES

The function of a child's shoe is protection, both from cold temperature and from trauma in the environment. Because of this, when neither of these conditions appears imminent, the normal child will rapidly discard his or her footwear. This habit frequently persists throughout adulthood. Of interest is that in economically depressed or meteorologically advantageous climates, the majority of children do not ever wear shoes. Studies of their feet show that they have an equal number of foot problems as does a similar, shod population—or even fewer.

Before walking age, protection from foot trauma is not a consideration, and soft shoes or booties are appropriate for thermal reasons. Once the child begins toddling, then protection from trauma is a good idea, and any type of shoe that is large enough and that will stay on the foot is appropriate. The function of a high-top shoe is to stay better on a fat foot and not, as commonly believed, to "support the foot and ankle." If foot and ankle support is necessary for a pathologic condition, then specialized shoe modifications or orthotics are needed. An ideal type of footwear for a human being, from toddler to octogenarian, is the rubber-soled canvas sneaker or a variation thereof.

It is good to remember that babies and infants normally have some degree of ligamentous laxity and fat feet. In fact, a high arch should give cause for concern, since this may be pathologic cavus, indicating neurologic disease. Also important to keep in mind is the fact that a so-called "corrective orthopedic shoe" will not correct a flatfoot, a rotational deformity of gait, or an angular deformity such as knock-knee or bowleg. It is probable that foot discomfort in children is more commonly due to inappropriately prescribed shoe modifications than to any other cause. The ideal shoe for a child, then, is one made over a nearly straight last, since the child's foot is normally straight; one with a sturdy enough sole to resist puncturing; one that is soft enough to adapt to the individual foot's size and shape; one that is large enough to allow for some growth; one that is resistant to moisture from within or without; and one that is economically sensible.

References

Metatarsus Varus

Bleck EE: Metatarsus adductus: Classification and relationship to outcomes of treatment. J Pediatr Orthop 3:2, 1983.

Kite JH: Congenital metatarsus varus. J Bone Joint Surg 49A:388, 1967.

Lichtblau S: Section of the abductor hallucis tendon for correction of metatarsus varus deformity. Clin Orthop 110:227, 1975.

Ponseti IV and Becker JR: Congenital metatarsus adductus: The results of treatment. J Bone Joint Surg 48A:702, 1966.

Rushforth GF: The natural history of hooked forefront. J Bone Joint Surg 60B:530, 1978.

Clubfoot

Gray DH and Katz JM: A histochemical study of muscle in clubfoot. J Bone Joint Surg 63B:417, 1981.

Handelsman JE and Badalemente MA: Neuromuscular studies in clubfoot. J Pediatr Orthop 1:23, 1981.

Laaveg SJ and Ponseti IV: Long-term results of treatment of congenital clubfoot. J Bone Joint Surg 62A:23, 1980.

Lovell WW and Hancock CI: Treatment of congenital talipes equinovarus. Clin Orthop 70:79, 1970.

McKay DW: New concept of an approach to clubfoot treatment: Section I—principles and morbid anatomy. J Pediatr Orthop 2:347, 1982.

McKay DW: New concept of an approach to clubfoot treatment: Section II—correction of the clubfoot. J Pediatr Orthop 3:10, 1983.

McKay DW: New concept of an approach to clubfoot treatment: Section III—evaluation and results. J Pediatr Orthop 3:141, 1983.

Turco VJ: Clubfoot. New York, Churchill Livingstone, 1981.

Turco VJ: Resistant congenital clubfoot—One stage posteromedial release with internal fixation. J Bone Joint Surg 61A:805, 1979.

Medial Deviation of the Talar Neck

Bleck EE and Minaire P: Persistent medial deviation of the neck of the talus: A common cause of in-toeing in children. J Pediatr Orthop 3:149, 1983.

Flatfoot

Basmajian JV and Stecko G: The role of muscles in arch support of the foot. An electromyographic study. J Bone Joint Surg 45A:1184, 1963.

Harris RI and Beath T: Hypermobile flatfoot with short tendoachilles. J Bone Joint Surg 30A:116, 1948.

Rose GK: Correction of the pronated foot. J Bone Joint Surg 44B:642, 1962.

Scoles PV: Pediatric Orthopedics in Clinical Practice, pp 93–102. Chicago, Year Book Medical Publishers Inc, 1982.

Tarsal Coalition

Asher M and Mosier K: Coalition of the talocalcaneal middle facet: Treatment by surgical excision and fat graft interposition. Orthop Trans 7:149, 1983.

Conway JJ and Cowell HR: Tarsal coalition: Clinical significance and roentgenographic demonstration. Radiology 92:799, 1969.

Cowell HR and Elener V: Rigid painful flatfoot secondary to tarsal coalition. Clin Orthop 177:54, 1983.

Jayakumar S and Cowell HR: Rigid flatfoot. Clin Orthop 122:77, 1977.

Mosier KM and Asher M: Tarsal coalitions and peroneal spastic flat foot. A review. J Bone Joint Surg 66A:976, 1984.

Convex Pes Valgus

Clark MW et al.: Congenital vertical talus. J Bone Joint Surg 59A:816, 1977.

Drennan JC and Sharrard WJW: The pathological anatomy of convex pes valgus. J Bone Joint Surg 53B:455, 1971.

Eyre-Brook AL: Congenital vertical talus. J Bone Joint Surg 49B:618, 1967.

Hamanishi C: Congenital vertical talus: Classification with 69 cases and new measurement system. J Pediatr Orthop 4:318, 1984.

Silk FF and Wainwright D: The recognition and treatment of congenital flatfoot in infancy. J Bone Joint Surg 49B:628, 1967.

Toe Walkers

Egloff AC: Idiopathic toe walkers: A true clinical entity. J Bone Joint Surg 58A:726, 1976.

Griffin PP et al.: Habitual toe walkers. J Bone Joint Surg 59A:97, 1977.

Cavus Foot

Dwyer FC: Osteotomy of the calcaneum for pes cavus. J Bone Joint Surg 41B:80, 1959.

Dwyer FC: The present status of the problem of pes cavus. Clin Orthop 106:254, 1975.

Japas LM: Surgical treatment of pes cavus by tarsal osteotomy. J Bone Joint Surg 50A:927, 1968.

Steindler A: Stripping of the os calcis. J Bone Joint Surg 2:8, 1920.

Freiberg's Infraction

Braddock GTF: Experimental epiphyseal injury and Freiberg's disease. J Bone Joint Surg 41:154, 1959.

Wiley JJ and Thurston P: Freiberg's Disease. J Bone Joint Surg 63B:459, 1981.

Köhler's Disease

Cox MJ: Köhler's disease. Postgrad Med J 34:588, 1958.

Ippolito E et al.: Köhler's disease of the tarsal navicular: Long-term follow-up of 12 cases. J Pediatr Orthop 4:416, 1984.

Kidner's Disease

Kidner FC: The prehallux (accessory scaphoid) in its relation to flatfoot. J Bone Joint Surg 11:831, 1929.

Zadek I and Gold AM: The accessory tarsal scaphoid. J Bone Joint Surg 30A:957, 1948.

Sever's Disease

Sever JW: Apophysitis of the os calcis. NY Med J 95:1025, 1912.

Plantar Warts

Montgomery RM: Dermatologic care of the painful foot. J Bone Joint Surg 46A:1129, 1964.

Toe Problems

Cockin J: Butler's operation for an overriding fifth toe. J Bone Joint Surg 50B:75, 1968.

Diamond LS and Gould VE: Macrodactyly of the foot. South Med J 67:645, 1974.

Meyerding HW and Upshaw JE: Heredofamilial cleft foot deformity (lobster-claw or split foot). J Surg 74:889, 1947.

Milgram JE: Office measures for relief of the painful foot. J Bone Joint Surg 46A:1095, 1964.

Phillips RS: Congenital split foot (lobster claw) and triphalangeal thumb. J Bone Joint Surg 53B:247, 1971.

Sweetman R: Congenital curly toes. An investigation into the value of treatment. Lancet 2:398, 1958.

Taylor RG: The treatment of claw toes by multiple transfers of flexor into extensor tendons. J Bone Joint Surg 33B:539, 1951.

Thompson TC: Surgical treatment of disorders of the fore part of the foot. J Bone Joint Surg 46A:1117, 1964.

Hallux Valgus

Auerbach AM: Review of distal metatarsal osteotomies for hallux valgus in the young. Clin Orthop 70:148, 1970.

Inman VT: Hallux valgus: A review of etiologic factors. Orthop Clin North Am 5:59, 1974.

Luba R and Rosman M: Bunions in children: Treatment with a modified Mitchell osteotomy. J Pediatr Orthop 4:44, 1984.

Children's Shoes

Bleck EE: Shoeing of children: Sham or science? Dev Med Child Neurol 13:188, 1971.

Cowell HR: Shoes and shoe corrections. Pediatr Clin North Am 24:791, 1977.

7

Orthopedic Strategy in Other Specific Conditions

CEREBRAL PALSY

Cerebral palsy is a nonprogressive disorder of motor function, including movement and posturing, and is the result of an irreparable lesion in the central nervous system. The lesion occurs during the period of early brain growth, either prenatally, perinatally, or in the first few years of life. Although the brain lesion is static, the problem of cerebral palsy is dynamic for the child, changing with growth, with the child's adaptation to his or her handicap, and with treatment. The incidence of cerebral palsy in children is about one or two per 1000.

The most common causes of cerebral palsy include anoxia, prematurity, hemorrhage during pregnancy, a difficult labor, birth trauma, postnatal trauma, infections, and kernicterus. Infants who are products of a multiple pregnancy and those with low birth weight, as well as those who suffer neonatal difficulties such as anoxia or convulsions, have the highest risk of developing cerebral palsy. In the past, those with hyperbilirubinemia secondary to Rh incompatibility also have been at high risk to develop athetoid cerebral palsy. Now, through improved management, the incidence of this basal ganglia lesion has been markedly lowered. The risk

of cerebral palsy increases with a maternal history of infertility and fetal wastage.

Cerebral palsy has been classified neurophysiologically and anatomically. Neurophysiologically, patients may have the pyramidal type, which includes spasticity and rigidity; the extrapyramidal or dyskinetic type, which includes athetosis and tension athetosis; mixed types, including elements of both pyramidal and extrapyramidal involvement in the same patient; and, less commonly, a hypotonic type, which includes those who are ataxic or flaccid, or both. The anatomic classification includes quadriparesis, with involvement of all four extremities; diplegia, with lower extremity involvement more severe than upper extremity involvement; hemiparesis, with unilateral involvement more severe in the upper extremity; and the double hemiparetic type, with bilateral involvement.

In the pyramidal or spastic type, the characteristics are hyperreflexia and hypertonia. Clonus is common, and hypertonicity is most pronounced in the upper extremity flexor groups and lower extremity extensor and adductor muscles. Joint contractures are often present, resulting from muscle imbalance and shortening, particularly in an active muscle whose antagonist is weakened.

In the dyskinetic or extrapyramidal type, hyperreflexia is much milder, and involuntary aberrations of movement are seen. Such aberrations include athetoid and choreiform activity and dystonia (increased tone and decreased control of voluntary motion). Dystonia is also known as tension athetosis. Dyskinetic patients frequently have more severe involvement of their upper extremities than their lower extremities. The decreased muscle tone found in this type of cerebral palsy, combined with uncoordinated and uncontrolled movements of major muscle groups, frequently leads to poor sitting balance and often poor head control.

The mixed type of cerebral palsy contains elements of both spasticity and dyskinesia. Involvement is frequently asymmetric. Often, the spasticity predominates in the lower extremities, whereas extrapyramidal patterns are seen more commonly in the upper extremities.

The flaccid and ataxic types of cerebral palsy show interference with equilibrium control, hypotonia, and normal or hypoactive deep tendon reflexes. Nystagmus is also frequently present.

Several other problems are frequently found in association with cerebral palsy. The most common is mental retardation, which occurs in about two thirds of the patients. It is seen most often in those with quadriparesis and least often in both the hemiparetic and the athetoid types. Seizures have been reported in approximately 40% of patients with cerebral palsy, those with the hemiparetic type being at the greatest risk. Other associated problems include emotional lability, personality disorders, learning disabilities, visual defects (particularly strabismus, visual field abnormalities, and refractive errors), hearing impairment, disorders of speech, and uncoordination of swallowing and handling salivary secretions.

The assessment of a child with cerebral palsy begins with the history of pre- and perinatal events, particularly a detailed developmental history documenting attainment of the motor and intellectual milestones. Poor prognostic findings include substantial motor delay, hypoactivity, premature development of one-sided motor dominance, poor feeding, variations in muscle tone (either hyper- or hypotonia), and abnormal persistence of primitive neurologic reflexes. The differential diagnosis of cerebral palsy in early childhood includes mental retardation, congenital myopathies, metabolic and degenerative central nervous system diseases, peripheral neuropathies, and neoplasms of the brain or spinal cord, or both.

Treatment Strategy

The top four priorities of the patient with cerebral palsy, in order of importance, are: communication, performance of the activities of daily living, mobility in the environment, and, finally, walking. These priorities must always be kept in mind.

The goal of treatment is to achieve the highest potential of intellectual and physical function possible for the individual. Most children require a program of physical and occupational therapy, the use of appropriate orthoses, and properly timed, precisely performed surgery. The indications for orthotic treatment are to prevent deformity, to substitute for an absent function, or to protect a weakened part.

Surgical goals are to correct or prevent deformity, to improve muscle balance across a joint, to stabilize a joint, and to decrease energy requirements during walking. In general, it is most advisable to perform surgery after the patient is five or six years old, when he or she is old enough to cooperate with the physician and the physiotherapist. Procedures to prevent hip subluxation or dislocation should not be deferred, however. If multiple corrections are needed, it is best to perform these with just one administration of an anesthetic agent in order to minimize hospitalization and rehabilitation time. It must be remembered, however, that altering any one musculotendinous unit or joint may have a significant effect on the remainder of that limb, the pelvis, or the spine. Another essential point to remember is that results of surgery in the extrapyramidal type of cerebral palsy, particularly in those patients with significant athetosis, are not as predictably good as the results in patients with spasticity.

In the absence of fixed bony deformity, soft tissue procedures such as tendon lengthenings, musculotendinous releases, and tendon transfers are helpful in preventing or relieving deformity. When fixed skeletal deformities are present, osteotomies, combined with muscle-balancing procedures, can be of significant benefit to the patient. Postoperatively, use of appropriate orthoses can protect a good surgical result, and night splinting is often an easy and very effective way of preventing an unwanted deformity from recurring.

Lower Extremity Surgery in Cerebral Palsy

The most important problem in the lower extremity with cerebral palsy is hip subluxation or dislocation (Fig. 7–1). This is usually caused by adduction, flexion, and internal rotation posturing or contracture. When hip abduction is limited to 30 degrees or less, and hip flexion contractures exceed 30 degrees, most hips are at high risk of instability and will require release or lengthening of the adductor and flexor muscles or their tendons, followed by use of abduction orthoses and night splints. With advanced subluxation or dislocation, procedures involving bone, including femoral or pelvic osteotomies, will be necessary to maintain a located and mobile hip.

The most common knee deformity in cerebral palsy is flexion contracture. Substantial hamstring tightness is the usual cause. Associated hip flexion and adduction contractures and tight heel cords are the rule (Fig. 7–2). Knee flexion deformity of more than 15 to 20 degrees interferes greatly with walking but may also prohibit the successful orthotic control of the lower extremities necessary for facilitating transfer activities in nonambulatory patients. Knee flexion deformity is managed by lengthening of the hamstring tendons. When more severe contracture is present, further soft tissue release, serial cast treatment, or bony osteotomies may be required.

The most common deformity in the lower extremity in cerebral palsy is contracture of the gastrocnemius-soleus muscle group, producing equinus of the foot. Plantigrade feet (angled 90 degrees) are essential for stable standing, walking, and even enabling one to wear ordinary shoes and have the feet rest comfortably on the foot rest of a wheelchair. Treatment of equinus deformity with stretching exercises or serial casting is sometimes, but not often, successful. Usually, Achilles tendon lengthenings are required, followed by orthotic control and use of night splints to prevent recurrence. Valgus deformity of the calcaneus and, less commonly, varus deformity are frequently associated with the equinus (Fig. 7–3). Tendon lengthenings may be appropriate when the valgus or varus is not rigid. With rigid valgus or varus, bone surgery is necessary.

Hallux valgus (bunion) is not uncommon in cerebral palsy and is effectively treated with an appropriate surgical procedure, the McKeever arthrodesis, done at skeletal maturity.

Upper Extremity Surgery in Cerebral Palsy

In the upper extremity, orthotic treatment (other than to prevent contractures in the hand) is poorly tolerated and rarely successful, but surgery has an established role. Surgery is most beneficial in the spastic hemiparetic patient, even though these children have derangements of proprioception and stereognosis that will significantly affect hand and upper limb function. Once a child has

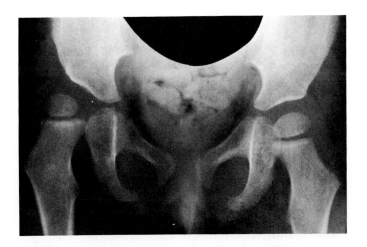

Figure 7–1. AP radiograph of the pelvis of a girl with spastic quadriparetic cerebral palsy, illustrating subluxation of the right hip and dysplasia of the acetabulum.

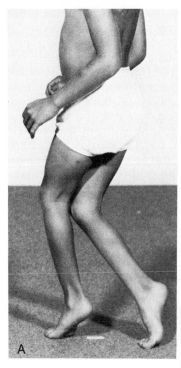
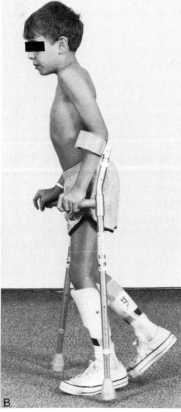

Figure 7–2. *A,* Gait photograph of a boy with spastic diplegic cerebral palsy. This is a common gait pattern. Note the flexion-adduction of the hips, the flexion contractures of the knees, and the equinus contractures of the ankles. *B,* In the early postoperative period, the patient is able to assume a more upright posture. Decrease in the hip and knee flexion contractures, plantigrade feet in floor reaction orthoses, and relief of his adduction contractures can be seen. He was soon able to discard his crutches.

reached school age and has developed patterns of hand usage, appropriate surgery can sometimes improve the function of a "helper" hand. It also can substantially improve cosmesis. The most commonly performed procedures in the upper extremity are those designed to improve elbow, wrist, and finger flexion deformities, decrease forearm pronation contractures, and improve opposition of the thumb.

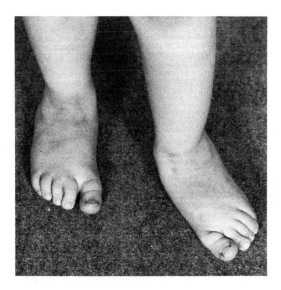

Figure 7–3. Equinovalgus feet in spastic quadriparetic cerebral palsy. This patient required arthrodesis of the subtalar joints and orthotic control to improve his gait.

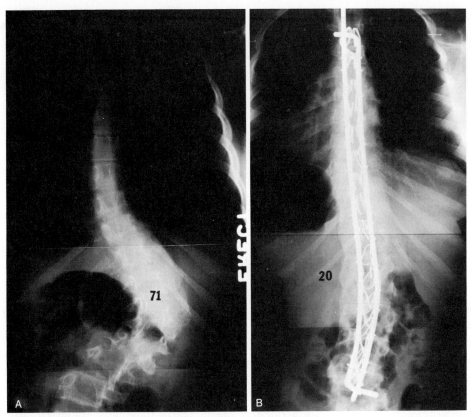

Figure 7–4. Severe right thoracolumbar scoliosis in a patient with spastic quadriparetic cerebral palsy. *B,* The scoliosis was treated with a posterior spinal fusion with L-rod segmental instrumentation and autogenous bone graft. Her spine is well balanced, and the curve has significantly improved.

Deformities of the Spine in Cerebral Palsy

Scoliosis, which develops in approximately 25% of the cerebral palsy population, is most commonly found in the quadriparetic group. Early recognition is essential in order to preserve spinal balance, walking or sitting ability, and respiratory function. In some cases, spinal orthoses can arrest or slow the progression of the scoliosis, but in many cases the curves will continue to progress, and surgery will be required (Fig. 7–4). Once a curve has reached 45 degrees, surgical correction with internal fixation and spinal fusion is usually indicated. Hyperkyphosis is not common in cerebral palsy, responds very poorly to orthotic control, and almost always requires surgery.

MYELOMENINGOCELE

A myelomeningocele is a sacular herniation of neural tissue and meningeal elements. It occurs most commonly in the lumbar, thoracolumbar, and sacral regions but may also be seen in the cervical area. A myelomeningocele is easily differentiated from a meningocele, which is a sac of meningeal tissues without neural elements, and rachischisis, which is the open exposure of a dysplastic spinal cord with no actual herniation (Fig. 7–5). Myelomeningoceles are often associated with hydrocephalus and with the Arnold-Chiari malformation. This can result in distal herniation of the brainstem or cerebellar tonsils, or both, through the foramen magnum.

The major musculoskeletal consequences are the result of the myelomeningocele itself. There is loss of motor and sensory function at, and distal to, the level of the lesion. With higher lesions in the spinal cord, reflex spasticity may sometimes be seen in the lower extremities. Otherwise, with low lesions, flaccid paralysis is the rule.

The prevalence of myelomeningocele is variable throughout the world, but the incidence averages one per 1000 births. This

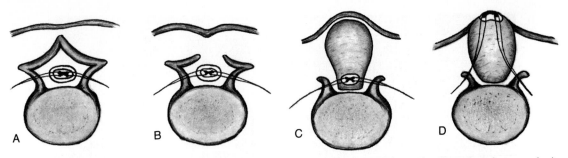

Figure 7–5. *A,* A normal spinal configuration. *B,* Spina bifida occulta. *C,* Meningocele. Note that the neurologic elements are normal. *D,* Myelomeningocele. Note the exposed neurologic elements and the marked anatomic distortion.

increases to 1 in 20 if one child in the family has the condition. Although the cause of myelomeningocele is unknown, prevalent theories hold that it is a multifactorial condition with an unknown inheritance pattern, probably modified by teratogenic agents and environmental factors. There are two hypotheses for the specific pathogenesis, one being failure of closure of the neural tube and the other being rupture of a previously closed tube. Recent advances in prenatal diagnosis, including determination of maternal serum alpha-fetoprotein levels, ultrasonography, fetography, and fetoscopy, have made prenatal screening and prenatal diagnosis possible with extremely high levels of confidence.

The diagnosis is obvious at birth, and assessment of a neonate with myelomeningocele includes general evaluation for specific associated anomalies such as cardiac defects, genitourinary and gastrointestinal anomalies, hydrocephalus with increased intracranial pressure, and brainstem anomalies. Evaluation of the spinal cord and peripheral nervous system and musculoskeletal evaluation are done as well. Lower extremity deformities are the rule with myelomeningocele because of congenital denervation, which leads to paralysis or imbalance of muscles in utero and subsequent contractures and bony deformity.

Before the use of the combination of antibiotics, surgical closure of the defect, and neurosurgical shunting procedures for hydrocephalus, few children with myelomeningocele survived beyond early infancy. Now, with coordinated multispecialty care, prolonged survival into adulthood is the rule, even for severely involved individuals.

The initial treatment of this complex lesion begins with early closure of the myelomen-

ingocele in order to prevent infection and to preserve function. If congenital kyphosis is present, it can be treated with partial excision to facilitate the closure. The next therapeutic step is shunting of the hydrocephalus, if present. Hydrocephalus occurs in more than 50% of these children. Next, attention to the urinary tract is essential. Programs of intermittent catheterization are now widely accepted and may be of significant benefit in protecting urinary function.

After the spinal lesion, hydrocephalus, and renal status have been stabilized, attention is directed at the musculoskeletal problems. The usual orthopedic strategy in myelomeningocele is to use preventive orthoses for spinal and lower extremity deformities as well as surgical procedures, such as soft tissue releases and tendon transfers, as indicated. Minimizing postoperative immobilization and recumbency helps reduce the incidence of osteoporosis and subsequent fractures, which are not uncommon in myelomeningocele patients.

Spinal deformities will develop in more than half the children with myelomeningocele. The most common deformity is paralytic scoliosis, although 20% of these children have congenital scoliosis with structural anomalies in the vertebral column (Fig. 7–6). Progressive congenital scoliosis cannot be treated by orthotic means, and surgical fusion of the structurally involved segments is mandatory when curve progression is documented. A few cases of progressive paralytic scoliosis may be treated successfully by orthotic means. A total-contact type of orthosis is most commonly used and is indicated for curves of 20 degrees or greater. Once a scoliotic deformity reaches a curvature of 40 degrees or greater, it is not controllable by an orthosis and should be stabilized by surgical fusion

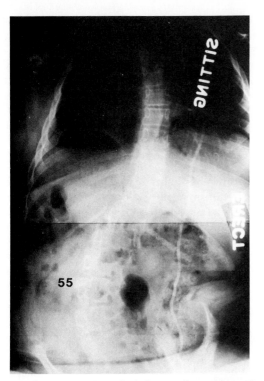

Figure 7–6. Paralytic scoliosis in a patient with myelomeningocele. The higher the level of the lesion in this condition, the more likely scoliosis is to develop. Virtually 100% of patients with lesions in the thoracolumbar region or above develop scoliosis.

with internal fixation and ample bone grafting. These curves require anterior and posterior spinal fusion. The recently developed technique of segmental spinal instrumentation has greatly improved the care of myelomeningocele patients with paralytic scoliosis. Of great importance is the fact that a tethered spinal cord or unrecognized hydromyelia may also result in rapid progression of paralytic scoliosis in myelomeningocele, and release of the tethering or ventricular shunting may result in the slowing or arresting of curve progression in some cases.

The problem of congenital or acquired paralytic kyphosis in myelomeningocele is a difficult challenge for a spine surgeon (Fig. 7–7). This lesion is never amenable to orthotic treatment and usually will require excision of the kyphosis with internal fixation and bone grafting, followed by orthotic support to attempt to prevent recurrent deformity.

Hip dysplasia and subsequent dislocation are common occurrences in myelomeningocele patients and are caused by muscle imbalance; in particular, activity of the hip flexor and adductor muscles with paralysis of the opposing extensor and abductor muscles

Figure 7–7. Clinical *(A)* and radiographic *(B)* appearance of kyphosis in a patient with myelomeningocele.

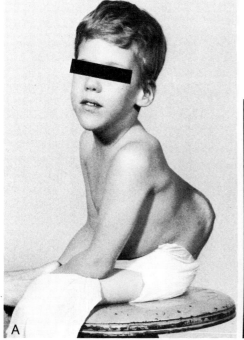

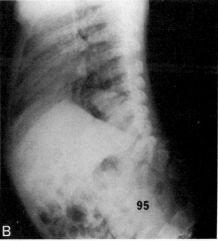

(Fig. 7–8). This is most often seen in children who have lesions in the mid- and lower lumbar region. The goal of hip management, above all else, is mobility and symmetry of the hips, regardless of whether they are dislocated. Early abduction splinting, followed by adductor release or posterior transfer of the adductor origin augmented by iliopsoas recession, may be necessary. Transfer of the iliopsoas tendon to the greater trochanter or transfer of the external oblique and tensor fascia lata muscles, or both, may also be indicated to stabilize a progressively dysplastic hip. For more severe hip involvement, open reduction, femoral osteotomy, and pelvic osteotomy may be indicated. Symmetric and mobile bilaterally dislocated hips are best left unreduced.

If functional walking is a realistic consideration, the knee must be free of significant deformity. If there is no fixed flexion contracture, orthotics may be effective, especially when supplemented by night splinting. When fixed deformity is present, corrective surgery is indicated, including hamstring release, lengthening, or transfer; selective knee ligament releases; or supracondylar femoral osteotomy.

Virtually every conceivable foot and ankle deformity has been described associated with myelomeningocele. When treatment is begun early, correction with the use of serial plaster casts and subsequent orthotic control may be effective. Deformities such as severe clubfoot, convex pes valgus, and calcaneus deformities require surgical correction.

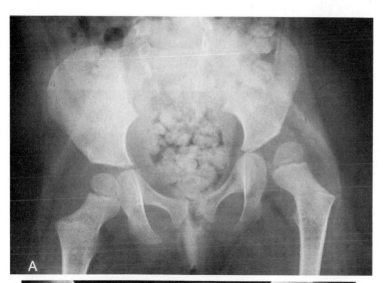
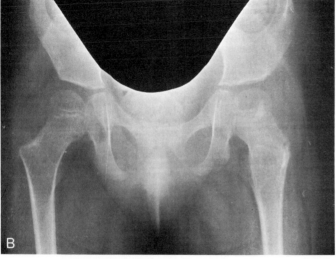

Figure 7–8. Hip subluxation and acetabular dysplasia in a patient with myelomeningocele. *B,* Following reconstructive surgery (including iliopsoas transfers), the hip has now stabilized, and the acetabular development has improved.

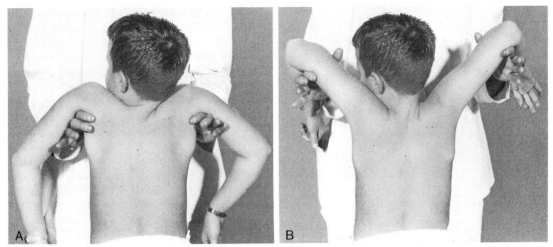

Figure 7–9. *A* and *B*, Demonstration of a positive Meryon sign (or "slipping through") in a boy with Duchenne muscular dystrophy. This is a classic sign of shoulder muscle weakness.

Throughout the management of a child with myelomeningocele, it is always critically important to remember the patient's intellectual, emotional, and social adjustment and family relationships as well. Many times, attention to these problems is equal in importance to the medical management—or even more so.

DUCHENNE MUSCULAR DYSTROPHY

This condition, also known as pseudohypertrophic muscular dystrophy, affects boys. Almost all cases are inherited as an X-linked recessive trait, with only about one third of new cases arising as spontaneous mutations. This shows the extreme importance of genetic counseling for a family with a child with Duchenne muscular dystrophy.

This disease presents after the age of walking, since the initial developmental motor milestones of head control and sitting are usually attained normally. The early gait is a wide-based waddle with increased lumbar lordosis. Initially, the heel cords are tight but not contracted, and the child never attains the ability to run. Shoulder girdle weakness is apparent. When one attempts to lift a child from under the axillae, a characteristic "slipping through" occurs, the so-called positive Meryon sign (Fig. 7–9). Another finding is the Gowers sign, which is the necessity for the child to use his arms to assist himself in rising from the floor (Fig. 7–10).

The natural history of Duchenne muscular dystrophy is quite similar in almost all cases. Progressive weakness develops throughout childhood, and the ability to walk independently is lost by most boys by the age of 9 to 12 years. During the growth years, progressive hip and knee flexion contractures, as well as equinovarus foot deformities, develop

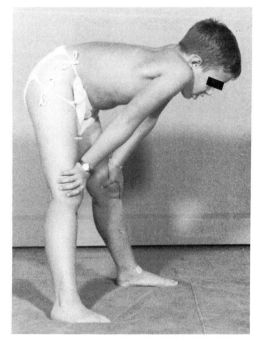

Figure 7–10. A positive Gowers sign in Duchenne muscular dystrophy. The patient uses upper extremity muscles to compensate for weak hip extensors in rising from the floor.

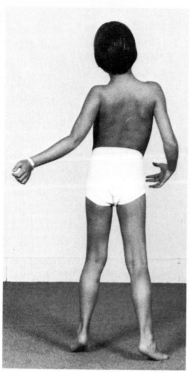

Figure 7–11. The wide-based gait of a boy with Duchenne muscular dystrophy. Note the hyperlordosis; the early, mild, right thoracic scoliosis; the use of the arms to maintain balance; and the pseudohypertrophy of the calf muscles and equinus of the feet.

(Fig. 7–11). Progressive scoliosis occurs in the majority of children with Duchenne muscular dystrophy, beginning after ambulation is lost. With progressive weakness and contractures and progressive spinal deformity, the patients ultimately become confined to bed. The last remaining functional muscles are the diaphragm, the muscles of swallowing, and the weakened intrinsic muscles of the hands and feet. Cardiomyopathy also occurs, and death, usually by the age of 20 years, is the result of either respiratory failure, pneumonia, or cardiac failure.

Physical examination of a boy with Duchenne muscular dystrophy shows proximal limb girdle weakness greater than the weakness in the distal musculature and lower extremity weakness greater than upper limb involvement. The gluteal muscles are involved first, followed by the quadriceps and then the foot dorsiflexors. Although the gastrocnemius and soleus muscles also become progressively weakened, they have a firm, rubbery consistency (pseudohypertrophy). The posterior tibial muscle retains its strength the longest in the lower extremity. Tendon reflexes are usually absent early in the upper extremities and the quadriceps, but the ankle jerk maintains its activity for a longer period of time. Intelligence testing shows that patients with Duchenne muscular dystrophy generally function slightly below average.

The most striking laboratory finding in this condition is an extremely marked increase in the level of creatine phosphokinase (CPK) early in the course of the disease. Values are usually several hundred times greater than normal. As the child reaches adolescence, levels begin to fall, and they may be only slightly greater than normal by the time of death (usually between the ages of 18 and 20 years in most patients). Other laboratory data include electrocardiographic abnormalities in 75% of the patients and abnormal electromyographic studies of skeletal musculature, typically showing small polyphasic potentials with increased recruitment of motor neurons during effort. Fibrillation potentials are also seen in the later stages of this disease. Muscle biopsy shows increased fibrosis, small groups of basophilic staining fibers, and groups of undifferentiated type 2C fibers.

Treatment should begin with genetic counseling and an attempt to identify the carrier status in related females. Seventy percent of carriers will show an increase in the serum CPK level, and an even higher detection rate is possible using phosphorylation of erythrocyte protein (Roses et al., 1976).

Although specific treatment for the involved patient is palliative, nevertheless prolonged function and perhaps a slight increase in longevity are possible. Early treatment is directed at preventing joint contractures by using physical therapy, such as passive range-of-motion and active resistance exercises. When walking is in jeopardy because of muscle weakness, bracing and surgery should be strongly considered and will almost always be extremely worthwhile. The goals at this stage are to keep the patient as mobile as possible, since ambulation using lower extremity orthoses can help prevent contractures and may also delay general physiologic deterioration, particularly the loss of bone mass and perhaps also the loss of respiratory function.

Surgical and orthotic treatment is indicated when walking ability is about to be lost. The treatment program may include subcutaneous release of some of the hip flexors and the tensor fascia lata muscle, if these are contracted. Knee flexion contractures rarely require surgical treatment and are usually easily managed by the use of serial plaster casts. Surgical treatment of the foot is almost always necessary; this consists of heel cord tenotomy or lengthening plus lengthening or transfer of the posterior tibial tendon to the dorsum of the foot. Surgery must be followed by immediate mobilization of the patient, since postoperative bed rest rapidly accelerates weakness and atrophy. Approximately three per cent of the patient's muscle strength will be lost per day if an individual with Duchenne muscular dystrophy is kept at bed rest. The patient should be standing in plaster casts or orthoses within 24 hours of surgery. Physiotherapy is resumed the day of surgery, and adequate analgesia must be provided.

Up to 90% of patients with Duchenne muscular dystrophy develop rapidly progressive scoliosis. Attempts at orthotic control of this spinal deformity have universally failed and may simply buy time while pulmonary deterioration progresses to the point that surgical treatment is not possible. Once the scoliosis curvature reaches 35 or 40 degrees, segmental spinal instrumentation is indicated to prevent collapse of the spine, interference with sitting balance, and increased restriction of pulmonary function. Such surgery is well tolerated by patients whose vital capacities exceed 30% to 35% of normal. These patients are easily managed on a Circ-O-Lectric bed, enabling them to be in the upright position within 24 hours of surgery and into a wheelchair by the third or fourth day. No postoperative cast or orthosis is required.

As the disease reaches its terminal stages, release of contractures may enable a patient to sleep on his back and may facilitate even the simple activity of rolling over at night in order to change from an uncomfortable position. Prevention of contractures and orthotic usage facilitate transferring the patient in and out of sitting positions. Even in the terminal stage, occupational therapy, devices to improve the performance of activities of daily living, and the use of oxygen at night to enable more comfortable sleep may benefit these unfortunate children.

MYOTONIC DYSTROPHY

This condition is also known as dystrophia myotonica or Steinert's disease. It is inherited as an autosomal dominant trait and is usually first noted in childhood or early adolescence. The first signs are often weakness of the hands and feet with stiffness and difficulty in releasing a grasp. Weakness of ankle dorsiflexion and knee extension also occurs, the weakness progressing from a distal direction to a proximal one. The classic facial appearance ultimately develops with wasting of the temporal muscles, drooping of the lower lip, and general sagging of the face (Fig. 7–12). Usually, the earlier the onset, the more rapid and severe the course of this disease. The myotonia decreases as weakness progresses and is potentiated by exposure to cold temperatures.

Myotonic dystrophy tends to be genetically enhanced, with each succeeding generation manifesting symptoms at an earlier age and having more severe involvement. Mental retardation is common, particularly in patients of myotonic mothers. Other associated findings include cataracts, testicular atrophy, infertility, and menstrual irregularity. Cardiac defects are seen in more than half the patients. It is important to know that these patients are also likely to be extremely sensi-

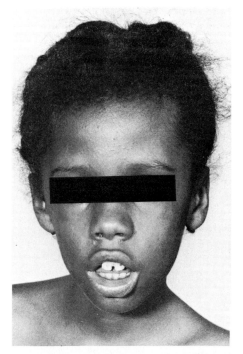

Figure 7–12. Typical facies in a girl with myotonic dystrophy. Note the drooping lower lip, the general sagging of the facial muscles, and the temporalis atrophy.

tive to morphine and barbiturates, which can excessively depress the respiratory center.

The diagnosis of myotonic dystrophy is based mostly on the clinical picture. The myotonia is often easily detected by means of percussion of the thenar eminence, which results in prolonged adduction of the thumb, and percussion of the tongue, which results in prolonged unilateral muscle contraction. Electromyography demonstrates the classic "dive bomber" pattern of waxing and waning myotonia. Slit lamp examination may show early cataract development, although this is unusual before adolescence. Electrocardiography shows conduction defects. Muscle biopsy is rarely indicated, but when done it demonstrates occasional internal nuclei and type I fiber atrophy.

The natural history of myotonic dystrophy is usually one of slow progressive muscle weakness. Many patients are unable to walk independently 20 years after the clinical onset of the disease. These patients most often live to mid- or late adulthood. Death is usually caused by cardiac failure or pulmonary infection secondary to respiratory muscle weakness.

Specific treatment for myotonic dystrophy includes exercises to prevent joint contractures and to maintain as much muscle strength as possible, orthotics for distal lower extremity weakness, and occasionally surgical stabilization of the foot to prolong walking ability (Fig. 7–13). Significant hip and knee contractures usually do not develop. Scoliosis

occurs in approximately 40% of patients with myotonic dystrophy but rarely becomes severe enough to require surgery. Orthotic control of scoliosis has been successful in this condition. Late in the disease, cervical muscle weakness, particularly in the extensor muscles, may warrant the use of a soft cervical orthosis.

CONGENITAL MYOPATHIES

These are a group of conditions—including central core disease, nemaline myopathy, myotubular myopathy, and congenital fiber-type disproportion—that present in an infant as a floppiness or hypotonia. The weakness is generalized but is more pronounced in the shoulder and pelvic muscle groups. Congenital myopathies either are nonprogressive or progress very slowly and are often inherited as autosomal dominant traits. They are best defined by use of histopathologic and electron microscopic studies.

The clinical picture of congenital myopathy often is a thin, asthenic child with muscle weakness (proximal greater than distal), hypotonia, and an elongated facies. Lower extremity muscle tightness and joint contractures often develop, and scoliosis is a common finding. The spinal deformity is almost always progressive, is poorly controlled with orthotics, and usually requires surgical treatment (Fig. 7–14). Patients with congenital myopathies may be particularly susceptible to malignant hyperthermia when exposed to certain muscle relaxants and anesthetic agents.

The natural history of most congenital myopathies is one of normal longevity, with independent ambulation usually delayed in childhood but maintained throughout life. Some cases, however, are unusually severe and may lead to an early demise from respiratory failure or infection.

ARTHROGRYPOSIS MULTIPLEX CONGENITA

Arthrogryposis means "curved joints." In this condition, there are multiple joint deformities present at birth (Fig. 7–15). Fixed contractures are secondary to failure of development of muscle tissue, which is replaced by fibro-fatty tissue. The cause is thought to be either degeneration or aplasia of anterior

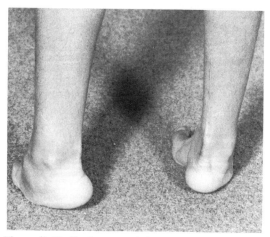

Figure 7–13. Equinovarus deformities of the foot and ankle in myotonic dystrophy. These deformities have recurred despite prior surgery and adequate orthotic control.

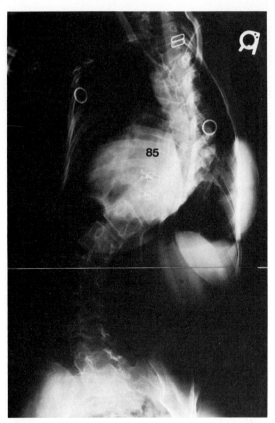

Figure 7–14. Severe scoliosis in a girl with nemaline myopathy.

This is a nonprogressive condition, always detectable at birth and commonly involving all four extremities, although only the upper or only the lower limbs may be involved (either symmetrically or asymmetrically). Characteristically, there is an abnormal fusiform configuration to the limb contour, thin papyraceous skin, atrophic subcutaneous fat, and absent flexion creases over the involved joints. Webbing may be present at the site of flexion deformities. Muscle wasting is severe, and active joint motion is minimal or absent. Sensory modalities and intelligence are normal in patients with arthrogryposis.

Scoliosis is common in this condition (40% incidence) and may stabilize with orthotic control, although frequently surgical fusion of the deforming spine is necessary. The hips are often involved with flexion and adduction contractures. These can lead to subluxation or dislocation. Extension contractures or even recurvatum of the knees is often seen, and severe foot deformities (most commonly clubfoot, but virtually any foot deformity) may be seen. Upper extremity involvement characteristically includes internal rotation contracture of the shoulder, extension contracture of the elbow, pronation of the forearm, and flexion with ulnar deviation at the wrist.

The treatment of arthrogryposis begins with an aggressive early program of passive and active assisted range-of-motion exercises for the involved joints. Occasionally, surprising improvement in range of motion and function can be noted, but this is not the rule. Protective splinting to maintain gains is worthwhile, and occupational therapy to provide improvement in performance of self-care activities and other activities of daily living is essential. Soft tissue surgery for severe contractures of the hips, knees, ankles,

horn cells in the spinal cord, perhaps due to an intrauterine viral infection of the central nervous system or to teratologic agents or toxins. Another etiologic hypothesis is that it is a primary muscle degenerative disease. There may be multifactorial causes for arthrogryposis. Sporadic cases are the rule, although there have been reports of this disease in siblings and in identical twins.

Figure 7–15. An infant with severe arthrogryposis multiplex congenita demonstrating severe bilateral clubfeet, recurvatum of the knees, and extension contractures of the elbows with flexion–pronation contractures of the wrists.

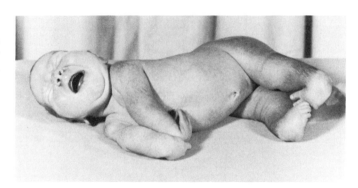

and feet results in a significant recurrence rate, even with subsequent splinting, and bone procedures such as osteotomies are frequently necessary. Osteotomies do not increase joint motion but may be useful in placing a limited range of motion in a more functional position. Talectomy is a classic and highly successful means of attaining a plantigrade foot.

It is essential for the parents and relatives of such children to understand that intensive physical therapy and prolonged orthotic treatment, often associated with multiple surgical procedures, will be necessary throughout the growth and development of the child in order to maximize his functional capability. Fortunately, these children are almost without exception very intelligent and resilient. Most become well-adjusted, productive adults. Longevity in arthrogryposis is usually normal.

FRIEDREICH'S ATAXIA

Friedreich's ataxia is also known as hereditary spinal cerebellar ataxia and is usually inherited as an autosomal dominant trait, although autosomal recessive patterns have been reported. Early clinical findings are usually noted between midchildhood and early adolescence and include an ataxic gait, problems with fine motor control of the hands, dysarthria, and nystagmus. Deficient vibration and position sense develops, and deep tendon reflexes are decreased or lost. Nerve conduction studies show decreases in both motor velocities and sensory action potentials. Cardiomyopathy is evidenced by myo-

cardial fibrosis and electrocardiographic changes. Progressive dementia begins shortly after the onset of the disease. The course of Friedreich's ataxia is one of steady deterioration, although occasional remissions or plateaus may occur. Most patients lose their ability to walk early in the third decade of life, and, because of progressive bulbar involvement, death occurs in most cases before the patient reaches the age of 40 years.

The musculoskeletal problems associated with Friedreich's ataxia are generalized progressive muscle weakness, severe equinocavovarus foot deformities, and scoliosis, which develops in more than 80% of the patients (Fig. 7–16 and 7–17). Orthopedic treatment is aimed at preserving joint motion by means of daily range-of-motion exercises and preventive orthotics or splinting. Later, surgical release of contractures and foot stabilization procedures are used in an attempt to prolong walking, to provide for the ability to wear shoes for comfort in sitting in a wheelchair, and to enable the use of orthoses for transferring the patient. Orthotic control of spinal deformities is indicated, but spinal fusion is often required to halt curve progression.

SPINAL MUSCULAR ATROPHY

This is a spectrum of diseases. At one end is a severe form that begins prenatally and rapidly progresses to death within the first year of life. At the other end is a very mild form with onset in late childhood or adolescence and a very slow rate of progression, associated with normal or nearly normal longevity. Regardless of its clinical form, spinal

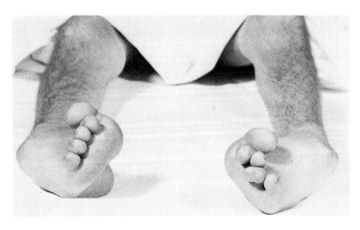

Figure 7–16. Bilateral severe equinocavovarus foot deformities in Friedreich's ataxia.

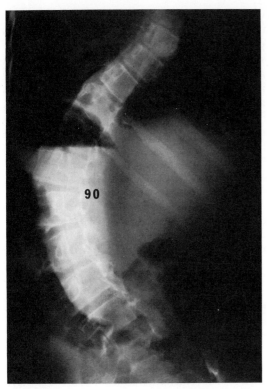

Figure 7–17. Paralytic scoliosis of 90 degrees in a patient with Friedreich's ataxia. Scoliosis occurs in approximately 80% of patients with this condition.

the knees are usually seen. Death usually occurs before the age of one year, although occasionally patients survive into early or midchildhood (Fig. 7–18). Because of their profound muscle weakness, patients with Type I spinal muscular atrophy are never able to attain independent sitting balance.

Type II is also known as chronic Werdnig-Hoffmann disease. This is a less severe form of the disease and is first detected late in infancy or shortly thereafter. Attainment of early motor milestones may be normal, but sitting is delayed, and most of these children never attain the ability to walk without external support. Type II is slowly progressive. The involvement of lower extremity muscles is more severe than that of the upper, and the proximal musculature is weaker than the distal muscles. Respiratory muscles and those innervated by the cranial nerves are less involved than with Type I disease. Deep tendon reflexes are absent. Progression in Type II spinal muscular atrophy may be extremely slow, and the development of lower extremity contracture is common. Preventive orthotic devices and splinting, surgical treatment of

muscular atrophy is inherited as an autosomal recessive trait. The disease is characterized by progressive degeneration of both the anterior horn cells of the spinal cord and the motor neurons of the cranial nerve nuclei. Sensory modalities are not affected. The spectrum of this condition has been divided into four types, Types I to IV.

Type I, also known as acute Werdnig-Hoffmann disease, occurs in approximately 50% of these patients and is the most severe type. There is a history of decreased prenatal activity reported by the mother, and there is little or no spontaneous movement at birth or during the first few weeks of life. Marked generalized weakness, hypotonia, and muscle atrophy are easily detected; deep tendon reflexes are absent; and fasciculations may be seen in skeletal muscles, as well as in muscles innervated by cranial nerves. The disease is rapidly progressive and produces great difficulty in swallowing, so aspiration is common. The cry is weak, and breathing is primarily diaphragmatic with intercostal retractions. Fixed deformities of the hips and

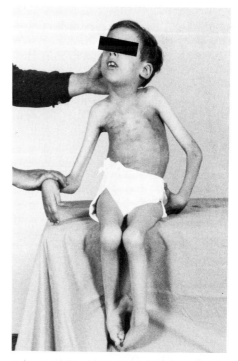

Figure 7–18. Child with Type I spinal muscular atrophy. Note the generalized atrophy of all muscle groups, the collapsing scoliosis, the equinovarus foot deformities, and the lack of sitting balance.

contractures and muscle imbalance, and orthotic or surgical treatment of the progressive scoliosis, which develops in all these patients, are extremely beneficial.

Type III spinal muscular atrophy is usually not detected until walking begins. The child has proximal muscle weakness and is unable to run or climb stairs (or has great difficulty in doing so). Some deep tendon reflexes may be present, but ankle jerks are usually absent. Lower extremity muscles are involved to a greater extent than are upper, and wrist extensors and intrinsic muscles of the hand are usually spared. The prognosis is excellent for long-term survival in this type of spinal muscular atrophy, although most patients will require a wheelchair by midadult life. As with Type II, nearly all patients with Type III spinal muscular atrophy will develop scoliosis. Orthotic treatment may occasionally arrest progression, but more often than not, spinal fusion is necessary.

Type IV spinal muscular atrophy is the mildest type, usually not diagnosed until the end of the first decade of life or during the second. These patients usually show very minimal proximal muscle involvement in the lower extremities and often no detectable weakness in the upper limbs. They always walk independently, and many can run.

The diagnosis of spinal muscular atrophy is suggested by the clinical findings and is substantiated by laboratory data. The serum levels of muscle enzymes are usually normal but may be slightly increased. Electromyographic findings are those of denervation with reinnervation and fibrillations at rest. Fasciculations and large polyphasic potentials are also seen. A muscle biopsy will show atrophy of both Type I and Type II fibers with occasional groups of markedly hypertrophic fibers. Fiber type grouping may also be seen.

HEREDITARY MOTOR AND SENSORY NEUROPATHY

This is a generic classification and includes several different types of peripheral neuropathies, such as Charcot-Marie-Tooth disease (peroneal muscular atrophy), Déjerine-Sottas disease (familial interstitial hypertrophic neuritis), and Roussy-Lévy syndrome (hereditary areflexic dystaxia). These have more recently been classified by Dyke into seven types of hereditary motor and sensory neuropathy.

While an in-depth discussion of each type is beyond the scope of this text, nevertheless patients with hereditary neuropathies have several features in common. The conditions are characterized by both motor and sensory involvement, although the motor deficit is much greater. The weakness is progressive, but longevity is usually normal. The inheritance pattern depends upon the type, some being dominant traits and some recessive, but sporadic cases of all types may be seen. Females tend to have more severe involvement than males.

The most significant neuromuscular problem for patients with neuropathies is weakness of the distal muscles of the lower extremities and associated loss of proprioception and interference with balance (Fig. 7–19). Progressive foot deformity is nearly universal, by far the most common type being equinocavovarus, although calcaneocavovarus deformity may occur. Most patients require early treatment, often consisting of the use of serial plaster casts and orthotic control, followed later by calcaneal osteotomy and soft tissue procedures or tendon transfers. Appropriate orthoses are needed to prevent or delay recurrent deformity. Triple arthrodesis

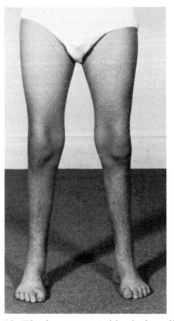

Figure 7–19. The lower extremities in hereditary neuropathy. This patient demonstrates cavovarus foot deformities, atrophy of the leg and distal thigh muscles, and a wide-standing base for balance because of weakness and abnormal proprioception.

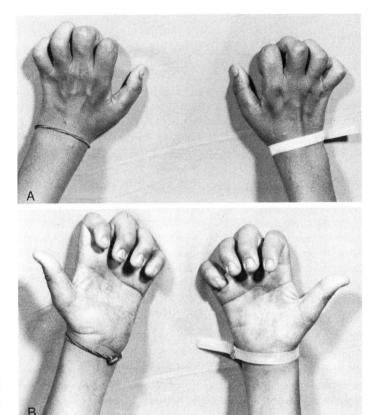

Figure 7–20. Dorsal *(A)* and volar *(B)* views of the hand deformities in a patient with hereditary motor and sensory neuropathy. Note the intrinsic muscle atrophy and the clawing of the fingers.

is the ultimate means of foot stabilization but should be deferred as long as possible, since long-term results are often disappointing, particularly in patients with sensory involvement.

Upper extremity weakness is manifested most often by intrinsic hand muscle involvement (Fig. 7–20). In some types of peripheral neuropathies, opponensplasty and other types of tendon transfer may be extremely beneficial in improving hand function.

Scoliosis and other spinal deformities are not common in patients with peripheral neuropathies. An exception is the patient with Déjerine-Sottas disease, particularly when the onset of this interstitial hypertrophic neuropathy occurs in infancy.

THE BATTERED CHILD SYNDROME

The battered child syndrome may be defined as the deliberate nonaccidental injuring of a child. It is the second leading cause of death in children younger than the age of six years. Approximately 80% of the cases occur in children younger than age three years. Battering happens equally to males and females.

The incidence of the battered child syndrome in the pediatric population in the United States is approximately one per cent. An estimated 1.6 million cases occur annually in this country, resulting in about 2000 deaths. This syndrome is responsible for 10% of all pediatric injuries. Approximately 90% to 95% of the injuries are inflicted by a parent, the father being slightly more likely to have been the culprit. Baby sitters and, less commonly, siblings also may be involved.

Characteristically, the abusive parent or family may come from any social class, although among unskilled and semi-skilled workers, the incidence is much higher. Several other factors are associated with the battered child syndrome. These include poverty, poor housing, unemployment, unwanted or illegitimate pregnancies, forced marriage, social isolation, youthfulness of the parents, lack of family support, social mobility, and excessive use of alcohol and drugs. Many of the abusive parents are the product of an unhappy childhood, and many have been the victim of battering in their own youth.

Only about 10% of the abusive parents suffer from a psychiatric disorder. Most of the remainder have long-term character defects and personality disorders and are not simply ordinary people reacting to unusual stress. The abusive parent frequently tends to have unrealistic expectations of the child.

The cause of the child abuse, then, is most commonly a triad of: (1) parents with the potential to abuse; (2) a special kind of child; and (3) a crisis, or series of crises, that precipitates the event. The parent usually has a low self-image, is unable to ask for help, and is very poor at dealing with stress. The abused child may be different, commonly being hyperactive or demanding or having a physical or emotional handicap. Many battered children were premature babies. The crisis that precipitates the event is often marital but may be related to unemployment or financial problems.

Failure to make the diagnosis and institute treatment may have severe implications for the child. Approximately 40% to 50% of the children will suffer repeated battering; 35% of these will be permanently injured; and about 10% of this group will be fatally injured. In addition, 30% of siblings are likely to suffer significant battering. Many battered children suffer permanent mental disturbances, including emotional problems or mental retardation, and many of these will become parents of the next generation of battered babies.

Medical Management

The medical management includes diagnosis, acute treatment, and protection of the child. Radiographic and photographic documentation is essential for the medical record, and reporting the incident to the police, social agencies, and the battered child management team in each hospital is mandated in all 50 of the United States.

The diagnosis begins with suspicion of this problem in children who present with any of the following findings: sudden or unexplained death; fracture or soft tissue injury; failure to thrive and signs of obvious physical neglect; and convulsions, drowsiness, or other manifestations of central nervous system disorders. The parental attitude or be-

havior is also of diagnostic help. Most parents show inappropriate behavior, either being very overconcerned or showing lack of concern about the situation, and they are often either overly patronizing or hostile. The history of the injury should be obtained separately from both the parents and the child, and the explanation must fit the degree of injury. Discrepancies and inconsistencies are common, and a history of the child being "accident prone, falling frequently, or bruising easily" should be viewed with skepticism. Delay in seeking treatment is also common in the battered child syndrome. Parents who abuse their children frequently make multiple visits to many hospitals in an attempt to avoid detection.

The physical findings in child abuse are signs of general neglect, skin and subcutaneous tissue injury, head and central nervous system injuries, skeletal injuries, and abdominal trauma. Signs of general neglect include pallor, malnutrition, "failure to thrive," poor body hygiene, and a repressed personality with flat behavior.

Skin and subcutaneous tissue trauma is the most common physical finding and may include burns (in 10% of cases), bruises, lacerations, and abrasions. These skin lesions tend to be clustered on the trunk or buttocks and also may be found on the limbs. They are often similar to the causal instrument, and lesions in different stages of healing are virtually pathognomonic for this syndrome.

Head and central nervous system trauma may involve lacerations and abrasions of the eyes, the ears, the nose, or the mouth. Scalp hematomas and alopecia may be noted. It is particularly important to understand that the violent shaking of a child can produce subdural hematomas or intracerebral bleeding secondary to tearing of the delicate vascular supply to the meninges and brain in young children. Such vascular trauma may produce mental retardation or a seizure disorder.

Skeletal system trauma in the battered child syndrome includes fractures, bony deformities due to malunions, limb length inequalities secondary to epiphyseal injuries, and occasionally unrecognized dislocations, particularly in the hands. The clinical signs of fractures are easy to recognize, namely tenderness, deformity, crepitation, swelling, and inability to use the limb.

Abdominal injury in the battered child syndrome is one of the two most common causes of death, along with head injury. Blunt abdominal trauma may produce rupture of the spleen, the liver, or a kidney, or tearing of other abdominal viscera with subsequent peritonitis or severe hemorrhage. The most common presenting signs of blunt abdominal trauma are vomiting, abdominal distention, tenderness, and hematuria.

The nearly pathognomonic triad for diagnosis of the battered child syndrome, therefore, is a child with a flat behavior pattern who has multiple injuries on multiple body surfaces. These injuries may be in various stages of healing. Color photographs of the entire child are needed for documentation for subsequent medical, legal, and social management.

Radiographic studies are essential in the battered child syndrome. A complete skeletal survey, or "baby-gram," is necessary, since bone trauma is the most common radiographic finding, occurring in slightly more than 50% of the cases. Twenty-five per cent of battered children will have multiple fractures, the ribs being the most common site, followed by the appendicular skeleton. A complete skeletal survey would include an anteroposterior (AP) view of the bones of the arms and legs, chest radiographs for rib detail, and AP and lateral radiographic views of the skull. Bone scans are not routinely helpful. Rib fractures are usually multiple and most commonly occur in the posterior or perivertebral areas. They may be due to blunt trauma or simply to squeezing or firm gripping of the trunk when the child is being shaken or thrown. The rib fractures are frequently in different stages of healing.

The appearance of a long-bone fracture gives substantial information regarding its cause. Direct blunt trauma produces transverse fractures with overlying soft tissue injury. Twisting produces oblique or spiral fractures of the long bones (Fig. 7–21). An extremely common fracture is the metaphyseal avulsion fracture; this is often pathognomonic for child abuse. It is the result of a sudden forceful jerk given to an arm or a leg, which results in the strong ligamentous attachments of joints avulsing small fragments of bone from the circumference of the metaphysis (Fig. 7–22). Such metaphyseal fractures occur in almost no other condition. This is frequently associated with periosteal stripping and subsequent subperiosteal hematoma. The periosteum in young children is very strong but is loosely applied to the bone and is very vascular. It is easily stripped

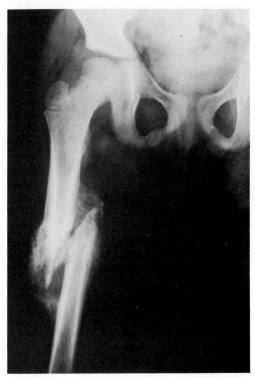

Figure 7–21. Spiral fracture of the right femur in a battered child. The fracture is healing in bayonet apposition. This child presented to the hospital for treatment two weeks after the fracture occurred.

when traumatized, and a large subperiosteal hematoma then occurs. After 7 to 10 days, ossification begins, which is easily detected on radiographic examination. The information gained from radiographic assessment of fractures in child abuse cannot be overstated.

Substantial twisting forces are required to produce oblique or spiral fractures. The suggestion that a baby has fractured the shaft of the femur because the leg was caught in the rails of a crib is not only unlikely, but probably impossible. Diaphyseal fractures are common long-bone fractures in abused children. These injuries are exceptionally rare in infants without abuse. They may be seen in various stages of healing in other limbs. When one fracture is detected, it is important to look for others, both old and new. Old subperiosteal hematomas that ossify can produce widening of the diaphysis of the bone.

Skull trauma will present as fractures of the skull bones, widening of the cranial sutures, or, rarely, ossification of old intracranial hematomas (Fig. 7–23). Skull trauma is seen in approximately 20% of battered chil-

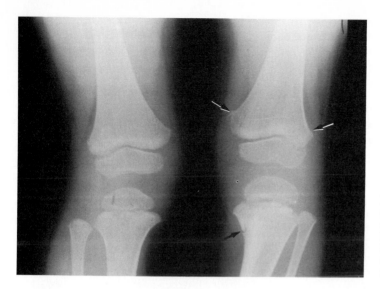

Figure 7–22. Typical metaphyseal avulsion fractures of the distal left femur and proximal left tibial in a battered boy. These fractures are produced by longitudinal avulsion of the metaphyseal attachments to the collateral ligaments of the knee.

dren. When neurologic signs such as drowsiness, convulsions, or others are detected, computerized tomographic scanning can be extremely helpful in assessing intracranial trauma. Spinal trauma is not common in child abuse, but when it does happen, it usually presents as a fracture or dislocation

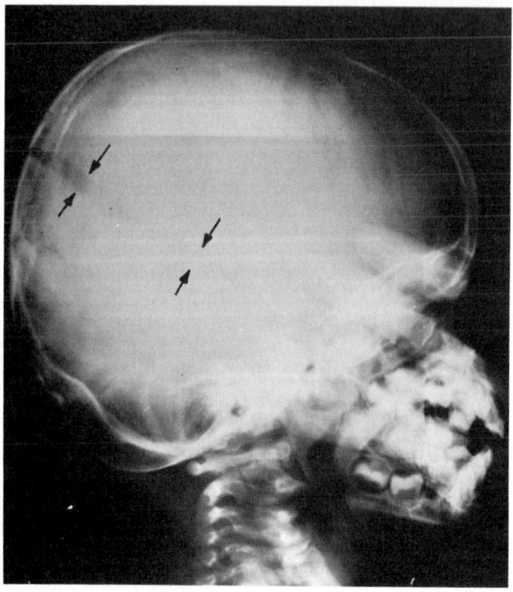

Figure 7–23. Linear skull fracture in a battered child. She was seen in the emergency room of the same hospital one week earlier for treatment of a fractured clavicle. The cause of that fracture was not detected at that time. Fortunately, she survived the skull fracture.

with anterior vertebral wedging and disc space narrowing. It most often occurs at the thoracolumbar junction.

The differential diagnosis of child abuse is not difficult to sort out. Accidental trauma is the most likely other diagnosis, and this can be determined, although sometimes with difficulty, by the child abuse investigation team. Other possibilities are much easier to rule out and include osteogenesis imperfecta, bone tumors, congenital insensitivity to pain, infantile cortical hyperostosis or Caffey's disease, blood dyscrasias such as hemophilia or leukemia, scurvy, rickets, syphilis, osteomyelitis, neurologic and muscular diseases, and the kinky-hair syndrome.

In summary, the management of a battered child requires (1) the care and protection of the child; (2) reporting the possible child abuse to the appropriate social agencies and the hospital child abuse team; (3) establishing with certainty the diagnosis; and (4) investigation and rehabilitation of the family and the family situation. The long-term management of battered children and their families is difficult and complex and is beyond the scope of this text. Ultimately, fewer than 30% of battered children will be mentally or emotionally normal, and fewer than 10% will have no mental or physical impairment. In the best of situations, approximately 80% of battered children will return to their homes by the end of the first year after diagnosis. A few will return later, but 10% to 15% will require placement in a foster home.

OSTEOGENESIS IMPERFECTA

Osteogenesis imperfecta is an inherited connective tissue disorder with an extremely heterogenous spectrum of types. The incidence of this disorder is about 1 in 40,000 births. Its specific cause is unknown, but the result is abnormal collagen in bone, ligaments, skin, the eye, and the ear.

Many classification systems for osteogenesis imperfecta have been devised; however, none has been accepted as the universal standard. Most patients tend to fall into one of three categories.

The most severe form occurs sporadically and is characterized by multiple intrauterine fractures, with severe deformities and bowing of the extremities seen at birth (Fig. 7–24). The limbs are markedly shortened. Many of these babies are stillborn or die during infancy, but a very few will survive into adulthood. The inheritance pattern of this form is most likely to be autosomal recessive, or it may develop as an unknown sporadic occurrence.

A second type of osteogenesis imperfecta presents with single or multiple fractures at, or shortly after, birth. These children have short limbs and a soft, thin cranium with bifrontal prominences that give a triangular appearance to the face. Most will develop flat or biconcave vertebral bodies, and more than half will have significant scoliosis develop during the juvenile years. The majority will be moderately to severely dwarfed and will have bowing of the long bones, particularly severe in the lower extremities. The incidence of fractures in this type tends to decrease after adolescence, because the patients either are more careful, are less active, or have some increase in the strength of their bones. Patients with this type of involvement also have defective dental development with thin enamel and soft dentin, thin papyraceous skin, easy bruisability, and increased ligamentous laxity. Fracture healing occurs at a normal rate in children but is frequently much slower in adulthood. Hearing loss is common in adults with this type of osteogenesis imperfecta. It is usually a conductive deficit due to otosclerosis involving the bones of the middle ear. Approximately 15% to 20% will become deaf in adult life. These patients have normal intelligence, adapt well socially, and usually become productive adults.

Children with the third type of this disorder may or may not show fractures in early life. Throughout growth and development, there is a small incidence of fracture occurrence. These children do not have long-bone bowing and are not dwarfed. The incidence of scoliosis in this mild type is no greater than that in the general population. Paradoxically, the incidence of blue sclera persisting into adolescence and adulthood is higher in this type. In this type of osteogenesis imperfecta, the inheritance pattern is usually autosomal dominant.

The genetics of osteogenesis imperfecta is variable. Most of the more severe cases are either sporadic or have autosomal recessive traits, and most of the mild cases are inherited by an autosomal dominant pattern. Assessment of the blue sclerae is a very unreliable means of predicting severity. In fact, many of the most severe forms are associated with white sclerae, and in others, the scleral

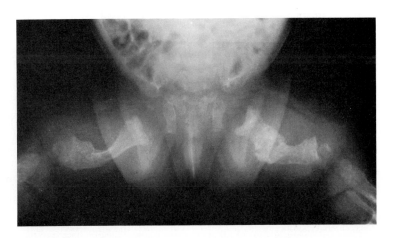

Figure 7–24. Severe deformities of the lower extremity skeleton in an infant with severe osteogenesis imperfecta. Note the widening of the bones and the healing fractures.

blueness varies with age, tending to decrease progressively. The exact cause of this disorder is unknown, but these patients appear to have a higher proportion of type III collagen, at least in their skin, than is normally found. It should also be noted that the milder types are more common than the severe ones, and that autosomal dominant inheritance patterns are more common than recessive or sporadic cases.

On radiographic examination, patients with osteogenesis imperfecta have changes proportional to the severity of the disease involvement. The cortices of the bones are usually very thin with notable osteopenia. Those with more significant involvement may have either very thin or very wide bones with bowing or other irregular configurations and often evidence of old or healing fractures. Bowing of the long bones is more severe in the lower extremities than in the upper. The skull is usually thin and may have a wormian appearance. In older patients, fractures do not heal as well, and delayed union or nonunion is common. Coxa vara and protrusion of the acetabulae are seen in those patients who are ambulatory and have the more severe type.

Orthopedic management of osteogenesis imperfecta is directed at appropriate fracture treatment. A significant advance in the management of severe long-bone deformity is intramedullary rodding. The indications for intramedullary rodding are frequent fractures of a specific bone or severe bowing deformity, or both (Fig. 7–25). Although there are problems, such as rod bending or breakage or erosion of the rods through bony cortices, and in many cases frequent revision of the rodding is necessary, nevertheless rodding can be of substantial benefit in minimizing bowing and fractures and in facilitating ambulation, not only through the growth period but also during adult life. Intramedullary rodding should be accomplished before the end of growth, however, since nonunions are much more common in adults.

When scoliosis develops in osteogenesis imperfecta, the onset is usually much earlier than one would expect with idiopathic scoliosis. Most curves are detectable by the age of six years. Once scoliosis becomes progressive and reaches 30 to 40 degrees, surgical treatment in the form of spinal fusion is mandatory (Fig. 7–26). Orthoses are almost completely useless in controlling spinal deformities in this condition and may simply serve to increase rib and chest deformity while the scoliosis progresses unabated. Although the vertebral bones are small and

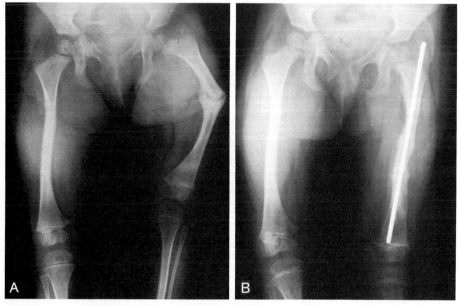

Figure 7–25. *A,* Recurrent fracturing of the left femur in a girl with osteogenesis imperfecta. *B,* Because of the shortening, angulation, and recurrent fracturing, an intramedullary rod was inserted to regain length and alignment and to decrease the incidence of fracturing.

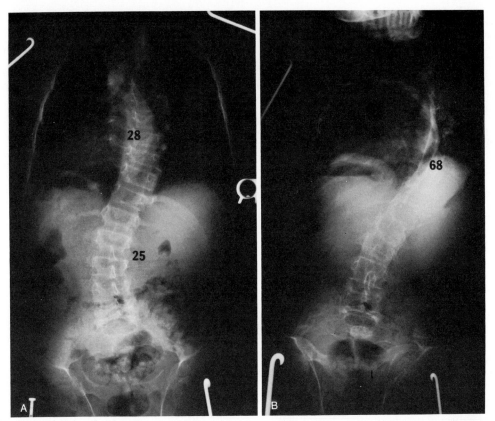

Figure 7–26. *A*, Right thoracic scoliosis of 28 degrees in a girl with severe osteogenesis imperfecta. Note the presence of intramedullary rods in all four extremities. *B*, Despite attempts at orthotic control, the curve progressed to 68 degrees. At that time, spinal fusion was performed.

soft, internal fixation can be accomplished with special-sized rods. The use of methyl-methacrylate to enhance fixation is often helpful. Even with a solid spinal fusion, how-ever, continued bending of the fusion mass may occur.

References

Cerebral Palsy

Bleck EE: Locomotor prognosis in cerebral palsy. Dev Med Child Neurol 17:18, 1975.
Bleck EE: Orthopaedic Management of Cerebral Palsy. Philadelphia, WB Saunders Co, 1979.
Gage JR: Gait analysis for decision making in cerebral palsy. Bull Hosp Joint Dis Orthop Inst 43:147, 1983.
Gage JR et al.: Pre- and postoperative gait analysis in patients with spastic diplegia: A preliminary report. J Pediatr Orthop 4:715, 1984.
Hoffer MM: Basic considerations and classification of cerebral palsy. American Academy of Orthopaedic Surgeons Instructional Course Lectures 25:96, 1976.
Hoffer MM and Koffman M: Cerebral palsy: The first three years. Clin Orthop 151:22, 1980.
Lonstein JE: Operative treatment of spinal deformities in patients with cerebral palsy. An analysis of one hundred and seven cases. J Bone Joint Surg 65A:45, 1983.
O'Reilly DE: Care of the cerebral palsied: Outcome of the past and needs of the future. Dev Med Child Neurol 17:141, 1975.
Thompson GL (ed): Comprehensive Management of Cerebral Palsy. New York, Grune & Stratton, 1982.

Myelomeningocele

Allen BL Jr and Ferguson RL: The operative treatment of myelomeningocele spinal deformity—1979. Orthop Clin North Am 10:845, 1979.
Asher M et al.: Factors affecting the ambulatory status of patients with spina bifida cystica. J Bone Joint Surg 65A:350, 1983.
Dorner S: Adolescents with spina bifida. How they see their situation. Arch Dis Child 51:439, 1976.
Drennan JC: Management of neonatal myelomeningo-cele. American Academy of Orthopaedic Surgeons Instructional Course Lectures 25:65, 1976.
Feiwell E et al.: The effect of hip reduction on function in patients with myelomeningocele. J Bone Joint Surg 60A:169, 1978.
Gross RH et al.: Early management and decision making for the treatment of myelomeningocele. Pediatrics 72:450, 1983.
Hoffer MM et al.: Functional ambulation in patients with myelomeningocele. J Bone Joint Surg 55A:137, 1973.

Lindseth RE: Treatment of the lower extremity in children paralyzed by myelomeningocele. American Academy of Orthopaedic Surgeons Instructional Course Lectures 25:76, 1976.

Menelaus MB: The Orthopaedic Management of Spina Bifida Cystica. New York, Churchill Livingstone, 1980.

Osebold WR et al.: Surgical treatment of paralytic scoliosis associated with myelomeningocele. J Bone Joint Surg 64A:841, 1982.

Rose GK et al.: A clinical review of the orthotic treatment of myelomeningocele patients. J Bone Joint Surg 65B:242, 1983.

Duchenne Muscular Dystrophy

Alexander MA et al.: Mechanical ventilation of patients with late stage Duchenne muscular dystrophy. Management in the home. Arch Phys Med Rehabil 60:289, 1979.

Brooke MH: A Clinician's View of Neuromuscular Diseases. Baltimore, Williams & Wilkins Co, 1977.

Drennan JC: Orthopaedic Management of Neuromuscular Disorders. Philadelphia, JB Lippincott Co, 1983.

Emery AEH: Duchenne muscular dystrophy. Genetic aspects, carrier detection and antenatal diagnosis. Med Bull 36:117, 1980.

Roses AD et al.: Carrier detection in Duchenne muscular dystrophy. N Engl J Med 294:1983, 1976.

Siegel IM: The Clinical Management of Muscle Disease. Philadelphia, JB Lippincott Co, 1977.

Siegel IM: The management of muscular dystrophy. A clinical review. Muscle Nerve 1:453, 1978.

Sutherland DH et al.: The pathomechanics of gait in Duchenne muscular dystrophy. Dev Med Child Neurol 23:3, 1981.

Vignos PJ Jr et al.: Predicting the success of reambulation in patients with Duchenne muscular dystrophy. J Bone Joint Surg 65A:719, 1983.

Wilkins KE and Gibson DA: The patterns of spinal deformity in Duchenne muscular dystrophy. J Bone Joint Surg 58A:24, 1976.

Myotonic Dystrophy

Brooke MH: A Clinician's View of Neuromuscular Diseases. Baltimore, Williams & Wilkins Co, 1977.

Calderon R: Myotonic dystrophy. A neglected cause of mental retardation. J Pediatr 68:423, 1966.

Carroll JE et al.: Diagnosis of infantile myotonic dystrophy. Lancet 2:608, 1975.

Harper PS: Myotonic Dystrophy, 12th ed. Philadelphia WB Saunders Co, 1979.

Lanzi G et al.: Myotonic dystrophy in childhood. Acta Neurol Bel 82:150, 1982.

Mossa A: The feeding difficulty in infantile myotonic dystrophy. Dev Med Child Neurol 16:824, 1974.

Congenital Myopathies

Drennan JC: Orthopaedic Management of Neuromuscular Disorders. Philadelphia, JB Lippincott Co, 1983.

Isaacs H et al.: Central core disease. J Neurol Neurosurg Psychiatry 38:1177, 1976.

Kurtenen P et al.: Nemaline myopathy. Acta Paediatr Scand 61:353, 1972.

Lenard HG and Goebel HH: Congenital fiber type disproportion. Neuropediatric 6:220, 1975.

Munsat TL et al.: Centronuclear ("myotubular") myopathy. Arch Neurol 20:120, 1969.

Ramsey PL and Hensinger RN: Congenital dislocation of the hip associated with central core disease. J Bone Joint Surg 57A:648, 1975.

Shy GM et al.: Nemaline myopathy. A new congenital myopathy. Brain 86:793, 1963.

Spiro AJ et al.: Myotubular myopathy. Persistence of fetal muscle in an adolescent boy. Arch Neurol 14:1, 1966.

Arthrogryposis Multiplex Congenita

Brown LM et al.: The pathophysiology of arthrogryposis multiplex congenita neurologica. J Bone Joint Surg 62B:291, 1980.

Drummond DS and Cruess RL: The management of the foot and ankle in arthrogryposis multiplex congenita. J Bone Joint Surg 60B:96, 1978.

Drummond DS and MacKenzie DA: Scoliosis in arthrogryposis multiplex congenita. Spine 3:146, 1978.

Friedlander HL et al.: Arthrogryposis multiplex congenita. A review of the forty-five cases. J Bone Joint Surg 50A:89, 1968.

Gibson DA and Urs NDK: Arthrogryposis multiplex congenita. J Bone Joint Surg 52B:483, 1970.

William P: The management of arthrogryposis. Orthop Clin North Am 9:67, 1978.

Friedreich's Ataxia

Drennan JC: Orthopaedic Management of Neuromuscular Disorders. Philadelphia, JB Lippincott Co, 1983.

Hensinger RN and MacEwen GD: Spinal deformity associated with heritable neurological conditions: Spinal muscular atrophy, Friedreich's ataxia, familial dysautonomia, and Charcot-Marie-Tooth disease. J Bone Joint Surg 58A:13, 1976.

Levitt RJ et al.: The role of foot surgery in progressive neuromuscular disorders in children. J Bone Joint Surg 55A:1396, 1973.

Makin M: The surgical treatment of Friedreich's ataxia. J Bone Joint Surg 35A:425, 1953.

Spinal Muscular Atrophy

Benady SG: Spinal muscular atrophy in childhood: Review of 50 cases. Dev Med Child Neurol 20:746, 1978.

Drennan JC: Orthopaedic Management of Neuromuscular Disorders. Philadelphia, JB Lippincott Co, 1983.

Evans GA et al.: Functional classification and orthopaedic management of spinal muscular atrophy. J Bone Joint Surg 63B:516, 1981.

Pearn JH et al.: A clinical study of chronic childhood spinal muscular dystrophy. A review of 141 cases. J Neurol Sci 38:23, 1978.

Russman BS and Fredericks EJ: Use of the ECG in the diagnosis of childhood spinal muscular atrophy. Arch Neurol 36:317, 1979.

Schwentker EP and Gibson DA: The orthopaedic aspects of spinal muscular atrophy. J Bone Joint Surg 58A:32, 1976.

Hereditary Motor and Sensory Neuropathies

Andermann F et al.: Observations on hypertrophic neuropathy of Dejerine and Sottas. Neurology 12:712, 1962.

Brody LA and Witkins RH: Charcot-Marie-Tooth disease. Arch Neurol 17:552, 1967.

Dyck PJ et al.: Peripheral Neuropathy. Philadelphia, WB Saunders Co, 1975.

Hagberg B and Westerberg B: The nosology of genetic peripheral neuropathies in Swedish children. Dev Med Child Neurol 25:3, 1983.

Karlholm S and Nilsonne U: Operative treatment of the foot deformity in Charcot-Marie-Tooth disease. Acta Orthop Scand 39:101, 1968.

Rossi LN et al.: Hereditary motor sensory neuropathies in childhood. Dev Med Child Neurol 25:19, 1983.

Steinberg D et al.: Refsum's disease—a recently characterized lipidosis involving the nervous system. Ann Intern Med 66:365, 1967.

Battered Child Syndrome

Akbarnia B et al.: Manifestations of the battered-child syndrome. J Bone Joint Surg 56A:1159, 1973.

Bittner S and Newberger E: Pediatric understanding of child abuse and neglect. Pediatr in Rev 2:197, 1981.

Galleno H and Oppenheim WL: The battered child syndrome revisited. Clin Orthop 162:11, 1982.

Helfer R et al.: Injuries resulting when small children fall out of bed. Pediatrics 60:533, 1977.

Kempe CH et al.: The battered-child syndrome. J Am Med Assoc. 181:17, 1962.

Osteogenesis Imperfecta

Albright JA and Millar EA (eds): Osteogenesis imperfecta. Clin Orthop 159:2, 1981.

Bailey RW and Dubow HI: Evaluation of the concept of an extensible nail accommodating to normal longitudinal bone growth. Clin Orthop 159:157, 1981.

Falvo KA et al.: Osteogenesis imperfecta: Clinical evaluation and management. J Bone Joint Surg 56A:783, 1974.

Jones CJP et al.: Collagen defect of bone in osteogenesis imperfecta (type I). Clin Orthop 183:208, 1984.

Moorefield WG Jr and Miller GR: Aftermath of osteogenesis imperfecta: The disease in adulthood. J Bone Joint Surg 62A:113, 1980.

Renshaw TS et al.: Scoliosis in osteogenesis imperfecta. Clin Orthop 145:163, 1979.

Glossary

abductor lurch Type of gait in which the weight of the upper body is shifted over the involved foot in stance phase to compensate for weak abductor muscles. This produces an abrupt sway or lurch to that side.

adolescent Defined in reference to scoliosis as any child aged 11 years or older.

anteversion An anterior twisting or angulation of the femoral head and neck away from the frontal plane of the femur.

apophysis A bony growth center, not a growth plate, that does not contribute to the overall length of a long bone. An apophysis usually has a strong muscle attached—for example, the greater trochanter of the femur.

arthrodesis The surgical fusion of a joint.

arthrography The radiographic imaging of a joint by injecting a liquid contrast material into the joint to outline its cartilaginous components.

arthroplasty The surgical reconstruction of a joint. This can range from simple excision of bone and cartilage to replacement of the joint with mechanical devices.

arthroscopy Visual inspection of a joint through a small telescopic type of tubular instrument, most commonly carried out for the knee or the shoulder.

arthrotomy Surgical incision into a joint. This is most commonly performed to remove a loose body or to drain an infection.

Blount's disease Pathologic involvement of the epiphysis, the growth plate, and the metaphysis of the proximal medial tibia, producing tibia vara or bowleg deformity.

calcaneus position Dorsiflexion of the calcaneus or hindfoot.

cavovarus Deformity of the foot characterized by a high longitudinal and medial arch with rotation of the hindfoot and usually the forefoot toward the midline of the body.

cavus An abnormally high longitudinal arch of the foot.

coalition Osseous or cartilaginous union of two bones of the foot.

Cobb measurement A means of measuring the magnitude of the spinal curvatures including scoliosis, kyphosis, and lordosis. The method is as follows: (1) Define the top and bottom vertebrae as those that tilt maximally toward the concavity of the curve. (2) Draw a line across the top endplate of the top vertebra and the bottom end-plate of the bottom vertebra. (3) Erect perpendiculars from each line if needed. (4) Measure the intersecting angle.

compartment syndrome Increased pressure in a muscular compartment that is completely surrounded by a fascial sleeve. This can cause necrosis of the muscles, nerves, and blood vessels.

Denis Browne Bar A bar used to connect two shoes together, usually used to treat rotational deformities of the legs or selected foot deformities.

diaphysis The shaft portion of a long bone, usually consisting of dense cortical bone.

dislocation Complete loss of contact between two joint surfaces.

distal Parts of an extremity progressively further away from the trunk.

dysplasia The condition of bad or abnormal development or growth.

epiphyseal plate The cartilaginous growth plate of a bone. Also known as the physis.

epiphyseodesis Surgical fusion of the epiphysis to the metaphysis of a bone by destroying the epiphyseal plate or physis.

epiphysis The end of a bone between the joint and the growth plate.

equinus Plantar flexion of a component of the foot. This can be the hindfoot, the forefoot, or the entire foot.

external rotation Turning of the anterior portion of a limb away from the midline of the body.

Fairbank test A test for pain or apprehension, or both, caused by patellofemoral instability. This is accomplished by attempting manually to displace laterally the patella into a subluxed or dislocated position.

forefoot   The portion of the foot distal to the tarsometatarsal joints. This includes the metatarsals and the phalanges.

hallux   The great toe.

hemimelia   Deficiency of part of a limb. When a complete limb is absent, the condition is amelia. Hemimelia can include many different deformities.

hindfoot   The portion of the foot that includes the calcaneus and the talus.

infant   Usually a child younger than the age of one year. When applied to scoliosis, however, infantile scoliosis refers to this disorder in a child aged three years or younger.

internal rotation   Rotation of the anterior part of a limb toward the midline of the body.

joint capsule   The ligamentous sleeve surrounding a joint circumferentially. Joint capsules may be attached to either the epiphysis, the growth plate, or the metaphysis.

juvenile   When used to refer to a spinal deformity, this refers to a child between 4 and 10 years of age.

kyphosis   A normal condition of roundback in the thoracic spine, the curvature being directed posteriorly. Kyphosis is abnormal when it occurs in the cervical or lumbar spine. The normal range for thoracic kyphosis when measured by the Cobb method is 20° to 45°.

lordosis   The normal anterior curving of the cervical and lumbar spines. Lordosis is abnormal in the thoracic region. The normal range for lumbar lordosis is poorly defined and depends to a great extent upon the orientation of the sacrum.

metaphysis   The portion of the bone extending from the growth plate toward the center. Each long bone has two epiphyses, two metaphyses, and one diaphysis. The distinction between metaphysis and diaphysis is an imaginary line.

midfoot   That portion of the foot distal to the talus and the calcaneus, but proximal to the metatarsals. These bones are the navicular, the cuboid, and the cuneiforms.

mobility triad   A term referring to the normal neonatal hip flexion, knee flexion, and hip adduction contractures.

neuropraxia   A condition characterized by interruption of nerve function, usually temporary and usually caused by trauma such as stretching or contusion of a nerve.

orthosis   An artificial mechanical device often referred to as a brace, utilized to protect a weakened part, to improve function, or to prevent deformity. An orthosis is not an artificial limb. An artificial limb substitutes for a missing part and is known as a prosthesis.

osteotomy   The complete division of a bone by cutting through it. Osteotomies are usually performed to change the angulation or rotation of a bone, or the position of a joint.

patella alta   A "high riding" patella, whereby the patella is located more proximally than normal.

patella baja   A "low riding" patella, whereby the patella is positioned more distally than normal.

physis   The growth plate or epiphyseal plate of a bone. Most long bones have one at either end, with the exception of such bones as the metacarpals or the metatarsals.

pollicization   Creation or repositioning of a digit in order to have it function as a thumb.

pronation   A term denoting rotation, usually of either the forearm, the wrist and hand, or the foot. It consists of rotating the anterior surface of the part toward the midline of the body.

prosthesis   An artificial substitute for a missing part of a limb.

proximal   The portion of a limb closer to the trunk.

pseudarthrosis   Literally "false joint," usually used when an attempted arthrodesis, for example in the spine, has failed to heal into solid bone and remains as an area of usually undesirable motion. Both sides of a pseudarthrosis may be covered with cartilage.

pseudoparalysis   The voluntary or involuntary guarding or failure to move a limb in order to protect the limb or to prevent pain.

ray   A term applied to the hand or foot describing the phalanges and the metacarpal or metatarsal bone and attached soft tissue.

retroversion   The opposite of anteversion. This term refers to a posterior rotation of the femoral head and neck relative to the frontal plane of the femoral shaft.

scoliosis   Lateral deviation of the spinal column caused by progressive tilting of individual vertebral bodies, usually accompanied by rotation of those vertebral bodies around their long axes. The rotation in true structural scoliosis causes deviation of the posterior elements of the vertebra toward the midline and of the vertebral body away from the midline.

spica cast Any cast that includes at least one extremity and the trunk.

spondylolisthesis Forward slipping of one vertebral body relative to the vertebra immediately below it.

spondylolysis A defect in the bony pars interarticularis of a vertebra.

subluxation Partial, but not complete, loss of contact between two joint surfaces.

supination A term denoting rotation, usually of the forearm, the wrist, the hand, or the foot, whereby the anterior portion of the limb rotates away from the midline of the body.

synostosis The fusion of two bones, usually on a congenital basis.

synovitis Inflammation of the synovial lining of a joint. This is usually associated with pain, swelling, and guarding.

Thomas test A test for hip flexion contracture performed by flexing the nontested hip maximally in order to stabilize the pelvis and then allowing gravity extension of the tested hip to its limit.

tibial torsion A twisting of the tibial shaft, normally inward at birth and progressing outward during growth.

torus fracture A nondisplaced fracture, usually through the metaphysis of a bone, characterized by buckling of the cortex.

Trendelenburg test A test for hip abductor muscle strength. When the patient stands on a tested limb, the normal hip abductors on that side will elevate the contralateral pelvis to maintain balance. The normal situation is called a negative test result. A positive test result shows dropping of the contralateral pelvis secondary to weakness of the tested hip abductors, resulting in the necessity to lean the upper body toward the tested side to maintain balance.

triple arthrodesis Fusion of the talonavicular, talocalcaneal, and calcaneocuboid joints of the foot, usually to correct deformity.

valgus Angulation within a bone, or of an entire bone distal to a joint, away from the midline of the body.

varus Angulation within a bone, or of an entire bone distal to a joint, toward the midline of the body. For example, "genu valgus" refers to angulation of the bone distal to the knee away from the midline, producing knock-knee. Genu varus, therefore, produces bowleg.

volar The anterior or palmar surface of the hand.

Index

Note: Numbers in *italics* refer to illustrations; numbers followed by (t) indicate tables.

MAJOR PROBLEMS IN CLINICAL PEDIATRICS

MAJOR PROBLEMS IN CLINICAL PEDIATRICS (MPCP)—
A series of important monographs focusing on significant topics of current interest. Unsurpassed in clarity and depth of coverage, each hardbound volume in the series covers a specific issue or disease, a recent advance in clinical therapeutics, or a newly developed diagnostic technique. A "mini-library" in itself, MPCP features concisely written, postgraduate-level information from highly-qualified authors.

Join the MPCP Subscriber Plan. You'll receive each new volume in the series upon publication—three to five titles publish each year—and you'll save postage and handling costs! Or you may order MPCP titles individually. If not completely satisfied with any volume, you may return it with the invoice within 30 days at no further obligation.

Timely, in-depth coverage you can count on . . . Enroll in the Subscriber Plan for MAJOR PROBLEMS IN CLINICAL PEDIATRICS today!

Available from your bookstore or the publisher.

Complete and Mail Today!

☑ **YES!** Enroll me in the **MAJOR PROBLEMS IN CLINICAL PEDIATRICS** Subscriber Plan so that I may receive future titles in the series immediately upon publication, and save postage and handling costs! If not completely satisfied with any volume, I may return it with the invoice within 30 days at no further obligation.

Name_____

Address_____

City_____State_____Zip_____

☐ Credit my salesman

Printed in USA.   283   PM2416D   Postage & handling additional outside USA.   00154

|||| ||

BUSINESS REPLY MAIL
FIRST CLASS   PERMIT NO. 5152   NEW YORK, NEW YORK

POSTAGE WILL BE PAID BY ADDRESSEE

CBS Educational & Professional Publishing
W.B Saunders Company
Order Fulfillment Department
383 Madison Avenue
New York, NY 10017